Your Ideal Cat

*Insights into Breed and
Gender Differences in
Cat Behavior*

D1057577

Your Ideal Cat

Insights into Breed and Gender Differences in Cat Behavior

Benjamin L. Hart, DVM, PhD
Lynette A. Hart, PhD

PURDUE UNIVERSITY PRESS
West Lafayette, Indiana

Library of Congress Cataloging-in-Publication Data

Hart, Benjamin L.
  Your ideal cat : insights into breed and gender differences in
cat behavior / Benjamin L. Hart, DVM, PhD, and Lynette A.
Hart, PhD.
      pages cm.—(New directions in the human-animal bond)
  Includes bibliographical references and index.
  ISBN 978-1-55753-648-8 (pbk. : alk. paper)—ISBN 978-1-
61249-255-1 (epdf)—ISBN 978-1-61249-256-8 (epub)
  1. Cats—Behavior. 2. Cat breeds. I. Hart, Lynette A. II. Title.
  SF446.5.H373 2013
  636.8—dc23
                          2012034713

Cover and interior illustrations by Emma Mooring

Contents

Preface

Kittens are such winning creatures that we can't help falling in love with them. But if you are thinking of welcoming a new kitten or cat into your home, do not underestimate the careful consideration needed to make your selection. The kitten you choose today will grow into the cat that could be your companion for the next fifteen to twenty years.

A number of experiences and thoughts come to mind in selecting a kitten. You may have really loved a Siamese you once had, but the vocalization may have been a bit too much, and perhaps he got into urine marking. A cat breeder you know may extol the virtues of the Ragdoll, another popular breed. Your cousin has fallen in love with the wild looks of the Bengal. Can a sampling of friends give you enough information about all of the main breeds of cats? And how can you evaluate the books that discuss the good points of the various breeds? The truth is, no one person can be the sole authority on all breeds. Breeders may have a bias, or at least a loyalty, toward their own breeds. Likewise, authors writing about certain breeds undoubtedly have their own biases.

The purpose of this book is to help you, the prospective kitten or adult cat caregiver (owner), select the breed, or breed type, and gender—neutered male or spayed female—best suited to your personality, other family members, and your environment, whether an apartment, a condominium, or a suburban home. A hastily made uninformed decision based on seeing a cute kitten might lead to an unhappy relationship with your cat. By carefully choosing a breed and gender using the information in the behavioral profiles provided in this book, you can anticipate a happy and loving long-term relationship with your new feline family member. For those of you who already own a cat, or who have established a breed loyalty, the behavioral profiles can still offer useful information for understanding the vagaries of cat behavior.

Naturally, people partially choose a cat because of its size, hair coat, or distinctive coloration. But the main reason for choosing a particular feline companion should be its behavior. We, the authors, are behavioral scientists who believe in giving advice that is based on data and sound reasoning. The rationale and methodology used to obtain the information provided in this book have been established, and the information is scientifically accurate and presented in a readily understandable format.

Before discussing behavioral traits and breed differences, we include chapters on how to use the information provided to select a feline companion (Chapter 1), choosing and welcoming your new cat (Chapter 2), behavioral differences between neutered male and spayed female cats to consider during your selection process (Chapter 3), raising cats to emphasize good behavior and discourage problem behaviors

(Chapter 4), and the historical background of cats (Chapter 5). In Chapters 6 and 7, the main body of this book, we discuss the specific behaviors of breeds. The book is rounded out by a final chapter on some intriguing cat behaviors: why they purr, yawn, eat grass, and flip out on catnip.

In the spirit of making this book user friendly, we do not provide research literature citations within the text. However, we do provide an annotated bibliography that readers who want more information may find useful.

• • •

We wish to extend our thanks to the many colleagues that helped make this book possible. The data collection and entry from eighty telephone interviews to develop breed-specific behavioral profiles was the result of efforts by Dr. Gretel Torres de la Riva and Dr. Shannon Reed. Dr. Neil Willits of the University of California, Davis, Department of Statistics performed the data analyses and provided statistical consultation. Dr. Torres de la Riva also helped in the construction of the behavioral profile graphs and the behavioral trait graphs. Our office manager, Marty Bryant, helped to coordinate team responsibilities and provided copy editing. The editors and staff at Purdue University Press, particularly Kelley Kimm, Heidi Branham, and Charles Watkinson, brought their many talents into the final editing, design, and production phases. All of the artwork, which so accurately portrays the essence of the various feline breeds and behaviors, is the contribution of Emma Mooring. Special thanks are due to the eighty dedicated, and very patient, feline veterinary practitioners whom we interviewed for behavioral characteristic ranking of breeds and genders. These practitioners are in the unique position of hearing many cat caregivers boast or complain about the behavior of their cats. Without them this book would not have been possible. Financial support, making possible the collection and analysis of the unique data set on cat behavior, was provided by a grant (#2009-36-F) from the Center for Companion Animal Health, School of Veterinary Medicine, at the University of California, Davis.

Chapter 1

How to use this book to select your ideal cat

Let's say that you've decided you want a kitten, but you don't know what breed to choose, or whether to choose a male or a female. You read about special features of some breeds, such as one that is exceptionally affectionate—a real lap cat—and another that is hairless, but warm and friendly. Some of your friends may say that you cannot predict how a kitten will turn out—a cat is a cat is a cat. Others may tell you to just stick with a female, or a male, and you'll be fine. Consulting cat lovers can be confusing because you are bound to get differing opinions.

Ask your veterinarian, "What is the best breed of cat?" and you are likely to hear, "This question is impossible to answer, because there is no 'best' breed." A breed that might be ideal for someone who lives alone and is away at work most days is different than a breed that might be ideal for a family with children who can be expected to play with the cat daily. Some people want to avoid the heavy-duty grooming that some cats need; others place behavior high above grooming.

1

This book presents a data-based approach to describing the behavioral differences among breeds and shows you how to evaluate these differences to select *your ideal cat.* Also presented are some essential differences between neutered male and spayed female cats.

There are a number of considerations with regard to choosing your companion cat. Certainly you might consider body size, hair length, coat color, potential allergies of human family members, and whether you wish to get a purebred or a generic domestic shorthair (DSH) or domestic longhair (DLH). But while size and color might be important to you, we are convinced that the single most important factor contributing to the richness of your interactions with your companion cat is the cat's behavior. This book provides profiles of the behaviors that are of most interest to those wishing to choose a cat, such as affection toward family members, aggressiveness toward family members or other cats, activity level, litter box use, tendency to urine mark inside the house, and even tendency to go after songbirds, for those whose cat is allowed to venture outside. Because we want to enhance your appreciation and knowledge of feline behavioral traits, we have presented the behavior profiles in a readily accessible format that includes both text and graphs. You can see from briefly browsing through Chapter 7 that there are major differences among many of the common breeds, giving you the opportunity to create and select from among a short list of the best breeds for you, and enabling you to advise others on breed selection.

A good way to first approach selecting a cat is to consider the behavioral characteristics that are the most important to you. Some people might like a cat that is very affectionate, perhaps almost clingy, and that can be counted upon to welcome visitors, and even sit in their laps. Others might prefer a bit more of a wild streak. Almost everyone wants a cat that is reliable in using the litter box and that does not take up the nasty habit of urine marking in the house. By selecting a pure-bred kitten, you have some idea of the behavior to expect when the kitten matures. With the DSH or DLH there is much less predictability with regard to future behavior. Chapter 6 contains graphs that rank breeds on each of the following twelve characteristics:

Affection toward family	Friendliness toward visitors
Aggression toward family	Fearfulness of strangers
Aggression toward other cats	Litter box use
Activity level	Urine marking in the home
Vocalization	Furniture scratching
Playfulness	Predation on songbirds

Let's say you are especially interested in a high level of affection, a low tendency for aggression toward people, and good litter box use. You could go through the graphs on these three characteristics in Chapter 6 and select, say, the eight breeds with the most favorable rankings in all three lists. Then you could look closely at the breed profiles presented in Chapter 7 to further narrow the list of strong contenders.

Very important is the sex of the kitten, which is discussed in Chapter 3. Gaining an understanding of the differences between sexes alone can make this book well worth reading. Because such a high proportion of cats in our homes are neutered or spayed, the gender differences we discuss are all based on neutered males and spayed females. While there are definite differences between neutered cats and those left intact, especially with regard to males, the age at which a cat is neutered or spayed makes no difference in its behavior.

The breed information in this book is based on the rankings assigned by eighty male and female feline veterinary practitioners. These authorities are members of the American

Association of Feline Practitioners who see a variety of breeds and breed types daily and listen to their clients boast or complain about their cats' behaviors. The methodology used to determine these rankings is explained in Chapter 6.

It is essential to emphasize that the information contained in the breed profiles does not represent our own opinions; in fact, we are waiting until this book is published to choose our first cat. That said, we believe that no breed is inherently any better than another, but rather that there is a niche for each particular breed. Ultimately, what makes the ideal cat for you depends upon who you are. Different breeds are suited for different environments, personalities, and lifestyles.

Chapter 2

Choosing and welcoming your new cat

General principles for choosing a kitten

Source of the kitten

By far, most people looking for a cat think of getting the generic domestic shorthair (DSH) or domestic longhair (DLH), and they are often attracted to the idea of adopting from a shelter. Others may find an abandoned cat and want to take it in. Still others may be familiar with a litter of kittens that a friend or neighbor has and wish to bring one home. If you choose a cat from a friend or a neighbor's litter, and you know the mother, you can get some idea of how the kitten will behave as an adult. Unfortunately, with most cats available in shelters, and with those that are abandoned, you do not have the opportunity to observe the behavior of the parents.

It is no secret that the ideal source for a kitten is a healthy litter raised by an attentive mother in a household where good nutrition and kind treatment prevail. If a kitten's mother shows

5

signs of not being adequately cared for, it is likely that the kitten is also not well cared for. For all the appeal that rescuing a kitten from neglected treatment may have, this does increase the risk that the kitten will grow up to have some behavioral problems.

Litter runts

Most litter runts turn out fine, but a runt does stand a greater chance of having future emotional problems than do other kittens from the same litter. The runt may have experienced harassment by its littermates, and this could have an enduring effect on behavior. There is also the possibility of undernutrition, since a runt is less able to compete with its littermates for food.

Getting along with the dog

If you particularly want a cat that gets along well with your resident dog, you would be well advised to get your kitten from a litter that has had exposure to dogs from a very young age so that it is habituated to this sometimes strange and overwhelming canine stimulus. At least introduce your kitten to the dog as soon as possible. It is almost guaranteed that a cat will not be at ease living in a household with a dog if the cat is first introduced to dogs as an adult.

Orphaned kittens

Orphaned kittens are another consideration. When a mother cat disappears, or the kittens are removed before they are weaned, they may be deprived of important maternal interaction. Regardless of the amount of cuddling we may try to give, there is no substitute for the constant interaction between a kitten and a natural mother. The task of bottle feeding orphaned kittens is laborious, and therefore sometimes litters are split up to reduce the feeding burden. When this happens the kittens' interactions with littermates are also reduced. Orphaned animals raised without mothers, and without their littermates, have a tendency to be overly cautious, fearful, and aggressive as adults. Although this tendency is stronger in dogs than it is in cats, it is something to take into consideration. If you decide to go with an orphaned kitten, try to get one that was raised with one or more of its littermates and with as much human contact as possible.

Advantages of selecting a purebred

Since almost all purebred kittens come from breeders, you often have the opportunity to observe the behavior of the mother, sometimes the father, and maybe even members of previous litters. Of course we all know that purebred kittens come with a predictable set of breed-specific genes leading to predictable body conformation and hair coat. In Chapters 6 and 7 we reveal that purebred kittens also come with the genetic basis for quite predictable behavioral traits.

Age of adoption of your kitten

At what age should you bring a new kitten into your home from a breeder or shelter? It is generally agreed that the best age is around eight weeks because by then a kitten is socialized with other cats and with people, and maybe even with a dog, in its birth home. And eight weeks leaves enough time in the cat's early life for socialization in the new home with different adults, possibly children, and maybe a dog. While there is some flexibility with regard to the best time for adoption, the main thing to keep in mind is that if you have a home environment that includes young children, dogs, or other cats, you want to be sure that the adopted cat, as an adult, will be comfortable in the environment. Introducing a kitten to your home at eight weeks of age will more likely lead to the cat being at ease than would introducing a substantially older one.

Selecting a kitten from a litter

Sometimes, especially with a breeder, you have several kittens in the litter to choose from. This brings up the issue of kitten temperament tests. Temperament is generally a much larger issue in selecting a dog than a cat, but if you have the opportunity to select a kitten from a litter, this possibility may come up. There are no scientific studies that show that kitten temperament tests are reliable in predicting anything about adult behavior. There is simply too much development, from the standpoint of behavioral and physiological growth, for us to be able to predict the behaviors that a kitten will exhibit as an adult. That's not to say that within a litter the kittens will not differ from each other; they well might. However, it appears as though the behavioral differences apparent in kittens do not necessarily carry over into adulthood.

That said, when selecting a kitten, you cannot avoid finding some kittens more appealing than others. Although your initial impression of a kitten is not a very reliable predictor of its behavior as an adult, there is nothing wrong with choosing the kitten that you find most appealing due to its color, body size, or its behavior. As a matter of fact, we recommend this because you are most likely to bond well with a kitten that appeals to you.

What about conducting a battery of genetic (DNA) tests on a kitten to predict adult behavior? While a complete genetic behavioral profile is a ways off, we are convinced that in the not too distant future geneticists will start piecing together various tests that will allow those wishing to adopt a kitten to get a good idea, via genome analysis, of how the kitten will behave (e.g., activity level, aggressive tendencies, and degree of affection) as an adult cat.

A kind of evaluation that makes a lot of sense is to observe the behavior of the mother, father, and even siblings from previous litters. Because the mother contributes half the genes and is usually available, if you are looking at a litter, most of your attention should be focused on her. Consider her reaction to being held, brushed, and approached by strangers. Ask about any problems with litter box use. If the breeder says something like, "Well, we've had some problems, but mostly we have it solved," it should be taken as a warning. If the breeder says that they've had some problems with urine spraying, that too is a warning. Keep in mind that females are much less likely to engage in urine marking behavior than males, so if a mother engages in urine marking behavior, this should be a factor to take into account.

With purebreds, you might ask about the behavior of the kittens from previous litters. You might even ask to telephone the caregivers of these cats from previous litters. If what you discover about these siblings from previous litters matches what you're looking for, you will have the best genetic profile available for your prospective feline companion. Also, if you are looking at a purebred, ask about the health of the mother and father to determine if they have any medical problems associated with their genetic line. (See the breed profiles in Chapter 7 for breed-related disease predispositions.)

Adopting an adult cat

You may consider selecting an adult cat because it seems that there is less to go through by not having to put up with kitten play, such as being tackled around the ankles, or to worry about training a kitten to use a litter box. However, adopting an adult cat has its own pitfalls. An older cat may not adapt to your household as well as a kitten would. And, especially if you adopt from a shelter, the cat may have behavioral problems that you will not know about until you actually have it in your home for some time. You may discover, belatedly, that the cat is an inveterate urine marker, and that may be why it was available at the shelter. Or, it might be one of those cats with a weakened sanitary instinct for using the litter box. An adult cat also may show an almost irreversible fear-related aggressive behavior toward children, a dog, or even another cat in your family. Thinking that it may just take some time, you might keep the cat around for a month or two, only to find that it does not become accustomed or habituated to the new environment. An option would be to adopt from a shelter in which the personnel have obtained information about the cat's history. Keep in mind, however, that the person who relinquished the cat may not have disclosed problem behaviors because he or she truly wants the cat to be adopted. Another option is to take in a cat from a shelter on a temporary basis, getting everyone in your family, and the shelter, to agree that this is a trial adoption. After a couple of weeks, you should know if the cat is going to confront you with serious problems. Meanwhile, allow the cat to experience the full range of stimuli in your home, including exposure to other pets, children outside the home, and others that it may encounter on a regular basis. It could be that there is a dog in your home that makes it extremely difficult for the cat, whereas it could be a perfect companion in a home without a dog.

When you are considering adopting an adult cat, be it a DSH or a purebred, you should be well acquainted with its behavior. The problem with adopting an adult cat from a shelter is that you do not have the opportunity to observe it in its previous home. In an ideal situation you would be able to see the cat in its current home environment and talk to the family members. And if it looked like the kind of cat that would fit in at your home, then you probably would be safe in adopting it.

Getting a feline housemate for a resident cat

Many people who have one cat think that they should perhaps add another one as a companion, based on the assumption that cats get lonely if left alone. The caveat is that cats have an inherent loner streak in them that varies from cat to cat but which differentiates them from dogs. If you were to ask your resident cat if he or she would like a feline household companion, there's a very good chance that the response would be *"No, thank you,"* meaning that the cat is perfectly happy alone. As a matter of fact, the resident cat might feel pretty antagonistic toward the new feline family member. Adding a second or third cat is often the cause of problems, such as fighting or urine spraying. However, many situations in which a cat is brought into a household with one or more resident cats work out fine.

Bringing home your new cat

The principles here apply to bringing home a purebred cat from its birth home as well as bringing home a DSH or DLH from a shelter. The discussion is framed in terms of introducing a kitten to your home, but it applies equally well to introducing an adult cat to your home.

Probably the very first consideration is toileting behavior. The last thing you want is for your new kitten to be reluctant to use the litter box. Kittens and cats want what is familiar. You will want to find out how regularly the kitten uses a litter box. Assuming that the kitten is using a litter box regularly, and therefore is accustomed to the smell of a familiar litter box, as well as a particular type of litter, ask the breeder or shelter if you can have the old litter box in exchange for a new box.

And, ask if you can take home some of the soiled litter to use as starter litter, then continue to use the same type of litter. If you want to change litter type, do so gradually by mixing the old type with the new type. Keep in mind that as nice as a familiar smelling litter box can be, an odor that is too strong can be repulsive. Regular daily cleaning, including removing solids as soon as convenient, is recommended. Problems with litter box hygiene are dealt with in Chapter 4.

Another consideration is scratching behavior. Find out if the kitten is starting to use a scratching post (or board) and, if so, keep in mind that each scratching post has a certain odor or smell on it deposited by the glands in the feet that scratch it. This odor is what attracts a cat back to that scratching place over and over again. There is not only a visual mark created by scratching, but a chemical mark—a feline ID number, as it were. Therefore, whether adopting a kitten from a breeder or a shelter, ask to buy the scratching post that the kitten was using. This will be an important household furnishing that will help your kitten to feel at home, and your kitten will probably go to the familiar scratching post as opposed to the arm of your newly upholstered chair to work over those claws. Even in the home, cats repeatedly go back to the same scratching place because it helps to freshen up that important chemical scent mark that lets any cats wandering through know that this place is occupied—never mind that this is unnecessary. Problems that occur with scratching behavior are dealt with in Chapter 4.

There is value in thinking about ways to welcome your new kitten or adult cat into your home, as well as in choosing a cat that is a good fit for your home environment. Cats have a keen sense of smell, and by providing familiar smells in the all-important litter box and scratching post, you are helping your new kitten or cat to feel more at ease in its new home and also lessening the chances that it will engage in house soiling and inappropriate scratching. It will not be long before your new cat's favorite sleeping areas contain familiar odors. And cats often deposit their scent by rubbing their corner cheek gland on doorways, stairs, and walls, further marking their territory and helping them to feel at home.

Chapter 3

Behavioral differences between male and female cats

Many people who are considering adopting a cat may not realize the importance of considering whether to get a male or a female. Yet, as we discuss in this chapter, there are major differences in behavior, and the differences apply both to purebred cats and to cats you may obtain from a shelter.

Most people adopting a kitten are aware that males are more likely than females to urine mark in the house, and that, if neutered, the likelihood of urine marking is greatly reduced. However, keep in mind that even neutered males are much more likely to urine mark than females. Urine marking is seen in about 10 percent of males, whether they are neutered as early as 8 weeks of age or neutered as adults, even after they have taken up the habit.

But the issue of selecting a male or female kitten goes far beyond that of urine marking. In this chapter we provide more details on the essential differences between males and females. As throughout this book, males are considered neutered and females spayed.

In our telephone interviews, the feline authorities were asked to rank spayed females versus neutered males on the same twelve characteristics as they ranked the breeds. The question about gender differences was presented before the breeds were ranked, and the gender comparisons were independent of breed designation. The graph on page 17 covers the twelve behavioral characteristics, which are described more thoroughly in Chapter 6. The characteristics are as follows:

Affection toward family   Friendliness toward visitors
Aggression toward family   Fearfulness of strangers
Aggression toward other cats   Litter box use
Activity level   Urine marking in the home
Vocalization   Furniture scratching
Playfulness   Predation on songbirds

In the graph, the vertical axis represents the point at which there is no difference between neutered males and spayed females. When a horizontal bar extends in the male sex typical direction, this means that males are more likely to express this behavior than females, and the longer the bar, the greater the difference between males and females. When the bar is in the female sex typical direction, this means that females are more likely to express the behavior, and the longer the bar, the greater the difference.

Particularly relevant are the differences in friendliness toward visitors, affection toward family, and fearfulness of strangers, aggression, and urine marking behavior. Males outrank females in being more social, affectionate, and playful, and of course more likely to urine mark. Females outrank males in being more aggressive toward both cats and people and more fearful, and they have an edge in litter box use. The aggression toward family members may be variable, and the cat will likely be aggressive at times but not at other times. In

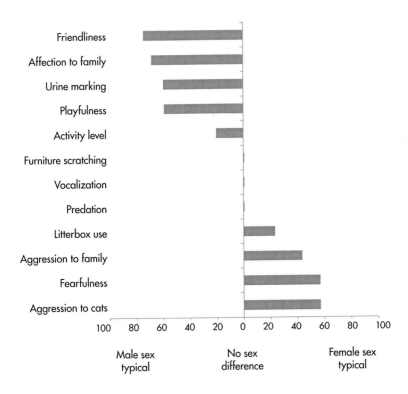

Graph showing behavioral differences between neutered male and spayed females. The vertical axis represents no sex difference. When the bar extends in the male sex typical direction, males are more likely to express this behavior; when the bar extends in the female sex typical direction, females are more likely to express this behavior. The longer the bar in either direction, the greater the difference between the sexes.

many instances, especially with young children around, a cat breed and gender with a very low tendency for aggression is the best selection.

Probably what most cat caregivers notice more than anything else is how affectionate their cat is. Whether you want your cat to be best friends with your child, or you want it to curl up in your lap, assuring affection from your cat can mean a lot. That said, affection is not tops on everyone's priority list.

Sociability is important when there are frequent adult visitors, or children coming over to play. A family cat that is friendly toward visitors—even strangers—is usually viewed favorably.

Lack of fearfulness of strangers goes along with being socially outgoing. When friends come to visit you, your cat can be outgoing and social with them, be indifferent, or be fearful and hide. For the most part, we like our cats to welcome our visitors, but if that is too much to ask, at least to not be fearful and hide.

Clearly the choice of gender can be a bit complex. Introducing a relatively nonaggressive and outgoing male cat to a multi-cat home has its appeal, but this could be asking for trouble because inter-cat interactions are the main cause of urine marking, which is the most common feline problem behavior for which veterinarians and other animal behavior authorities are consulted. Introducing the more affectionate, nonaggressive, outgoing, and playful male into a home where he is the only cat is less likely to lead to urine marking. Still, there are no guarantees. If urine marking does occur, keep in mind that psychotropic medications are available. (See the annotated bibliography for additional reading.)

Chapter 4

Raising kittens to emphasize good behavior and discourage problem behaviors

When raising a kitten we are logically concerned with its well-being and making sure its physiological needs are met. But keep in mind that time spent shaping your kitten's behavior is also a good investment in effort. Studies show that early learning experiences have more staying power than later learning experiences. In this chapter we discuss the important issues of litter box use; outdoor elimination training, for those cats with access to the outdoors; avoiding triggers for urine marking in the home; directing scratching behavior to an appropriate object; and encouraging friendly behavior toward children, and even dogs, by taking advantage of the early experience effect.

When it comes to behavior, there are two complementary approaches. One approach is to select a breed or gender that is ranked favorably on the behavior—not necessarily at the top or bottom, but at least midway in the desired direction. The other approach, discussed in this chapter, is to stage the environment in your home and monitor your own behavior to emphasize good behaviors and discourage problem behaviors in your cat.

Litter box use

One behavior that endears cats to us is the ease with which they can be housetrained. Just provide a litter box and commercial litter and the cat is trained. Keep in mind, however, that house soiling is not uncommon in cats and, in fact, is often a reason that cat caregivers seek professional help. Taking a look at what goes on in nature is useful.

Out in the wild, virtually all felids carry at least a light load of intestinal parasitic worms. These worms reproduce by depositing eggs in the stools. When the stools are a few days old, the eggs hatch into worm larvae that are infective to cats. These squiggly worm larvae latch onto what is passing by, and if the larvae are lucky the passerby is a cat. The larvae attach to the cat's hair and are then groomed off and swallowed, and the cat is then infected, or re-infected.

Cats living outdoors a lot of the day tend to have specific toilet areas, which have a bit of the smell of feces and urine that indicates a place to eliminate. These areas are away from sleeping and resting places. By going to the toilet area, digging a hole, covering the stool or urine, and then getting out of there, infestation with worm larvae is minimized. From the cat's point of view, the neighbor's sandbox is an ideal toilet area.

An established toilet area has a telltale stool and urine odor. Not an odor that we can easily detect, but one that cats, with an olfactory sense thousands of times better than ours, can. The indoor litter box, even when kept clean by our standards, smells clearly like a toilet area to the cat, and the cat is attracted back to that area for future business. If the toilet area is used too much, and fecal droppings are getting too concentrated, not only is the odor going to be very strong, but, in nature, infective parasitic larvae can become too numerous. The overused toilet area indicates to the cat a "parasite minefield." Extrapolate this to the litter box that is cleaned too infrequently: The cat does not want to use that toilet area; better to use the living room carpet in the corner. Never mind that the cat does not have intestinal parasites (which cats generally cannot feel)—the cat's instinct, from ancestors that almost always had some parasites, is to act as though it and other cats have parasites. Cats are instinctually guided by the odor principle; an appropriate toilet area should have a small bit of fecal and urine odor, but not a strong odor.

Additional litter box principles to keep in mind are that once a cat is accustomed to a certain type of litter or litter box, it is best to keep this consistent. In Chapter 2, on choosing and bringing home your new cat, we mentioned the advantage of bringing home the cat's litter box and some of the soiled litter as a "starter" for the litter box in the new home. If you cannot get the litter box, at least bring back some mildly soiled litter. (If someone says you are crazy, explain a bit—you may help the next person selecting a cat.) If a kitten just shows up at your door, it is useful to know that most cats have a litter preference, with the fine clumping clay litter favored most frequently.

If a newly acquired kitten is not using a litter box regularly, you can offer two or three types of litter, in different boxes, to see if one is preferred. Also, if you have a multi-cat home, do not expect all cats to use the same litter box. Just assume that the new cat will prefer its own litter and litter box.

Given the principles of toileting, attention to litter box hygiene is important in reducing the likelihood of inappropriate elimination. The litter box should be cleaned of all waste material at least on a daily basis; twice a day is the best practice. If the litter box itself becomes visibly soiled with feces it is necessary to wash the box. And do not make the mistake that some cat caregivers do by placing the litter box, food dish, and water bowl all together. Having to eat and drink right next to where one poops and pees is no more fitting for a cat than a for person.

If you are selecting a purebred cat it will be useful to know that some breeds seem to excel in ease of litter box use and some are known for being difficult. Known for being most difficult is the Persian, and known for being relatively good at litter box use are the Tonkinese, Burmese, and Russian Blue. Our authorities ranked the domestic shorthair (DSH) as the easiest in litter box training. Check out the rest of the breeds with regard to this behavior in Chapter 6.

Finally, when you have to deal with an "accident" or two, where a cat has chosen an alternative toilet area in the home, reevaluate the litter box principles and make using the litter box more appealing. Then, because residual urine and fecal odors indicate a toilet area, it is important to immediately clean the soiled area and make it unavailable to your cat (for example, by covering the area with plastic sheeting). Do not expect that just thoroughly cleaning will do the job; what looks and smells clean to us can still have a toilet-area odor to the cat.

Outdoor litter area

Cats that are expected to eliminate outdoors present a some-what different set of concerns. They can be encouraged to use one or two specific toilet areas outside by digging a shallow hole at least the size of a large litter box and adding an inch or two of sand. To further indicate that this is a toilet area, you could add some fecal- or urine-tainted litter to begin the orientation. Once it is being used, this area can then be cleaned and scooped out in the same manner as a litter box.

Urine marking

In expecting cats to use the litter box we are asking them to do in the home what they normally do in nature. In expecting cats to not urine mark some furniture or wall of the house, we are asking them to *not* do in the home what they normally do in nature. In nature, urine spraying by cats is a type of territorial marking, mostly performed by tomcats. Urine for cats represents a fingerprint, and cats can identify the smell of individual cats by their urine. By urine marking prominent objects in its territory, a cat familiarizes itself with its own territory and home range. The pervasive urine odor probably makes a cat more self-assured and comfortable, and it also communicates the cat's presence to other cats in the surrounding area. Cats do not mark the boundaries of their territory as one would put up a fence, but rather they mark prominent objects within the territory. Urine marking by females is also undoubtedly useful during the breeding season for attracting males wandering through their territory.

We use the terms urine marking and urine spraying interchangeably. While the spraying of a vertical surface, such as a wall, is by far the most common type of urine marking, sometimes cats use a squatting posture to deposit a bit of urine on horizontal items, such as the caregiver's clothes or bed linens. Clearly though, the cat is not finding an alternative to the litter box, which is still used for most urinations. One can even see urine marking on a horizontal object and urine spaying on a vertical object by the same cat. In urine marking as typically expressed in urine spraying, the cat approaches a vertical target, briefly smells it and then turns, lifting the tail, and

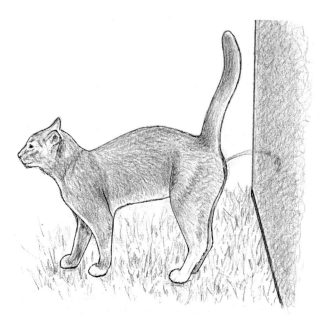

Urine marking, which is different than horizontal inappropriate urination outside the litter box, can be decreased by avoiding altercations between cats.

sprays a bit of urine on the vertical target; the urinary bladder is usually not emptied.

Because urine marking is primarily a male behavior, we mostly avoid the problem by just selecting a female or by neutering a male. Males may be neutered before puberty or as adults, even after they take up marking. If done on adult cats that have begun marking, neutering is effective in eliminating the problem in about 90 percent of cats. The extent of experience an adult male has in engaging in urine marking appears to play no role in whether or not the cat will be one of the persisting 10 percent. For males neutered before puberty, one can expect about 10 percent to take up urine marking in the house as an adult. While females are not found urine marking nearly as much as males, a few do take it up.

Here is another area where breed identity makes a difference. The DSH ranks at the very top in urine marking the house. The Bengal, in keeping with its wild miniature tiger persona, is second, followed by the DLH and Siamese. With a reputation for being least likely to urine mark are the hairless Sphynx, Cornish Rex, Ragdoll, and Burmese. Check Chapter 6 for a ranking of all breeds.

In raising a kitten, keep in mind that the onset of spraying is most often related to unfriendly or aggressive interactions with other cats. A common cause is the introduction of a new cat into the household. Sometimes cats can be seen staring at another cat through a window and getting upset. This could be a prelude to marking the house, and in some cases blocking visual access to outside cats is advisable.

In the home you should not let aggressive interactions between cats continue, especially if one of the cats is a male. Make arrangements so that the cats have their own living area with food, water, and a litter box. Don't wait for urine spraying to start up. Some caregivers have creatively created separate spaces with the use of a screen door. The cats can still see and smell each other, but not fight. If all goes well, the cats gradually can be allowed physical contact.

Inappropriate scratching

As some cat caregivers have learned, a mildmannered cat can make quick work of a nice couch or easy chair. However, this behavior can be directed to an acceptable site, usually a scratching post. As with litter box training, taking a look at what goes on in nature is useful.

Many outdoor cats have a favorite scratching tree that is prominent, and the cat repeatedly works over the trunk of this tree with its claws. Because of the scratched appear-

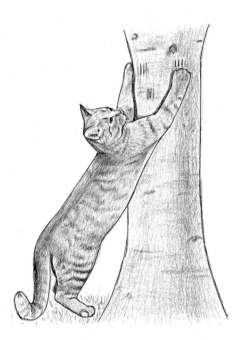

Scratching an object, especially a tree trunk, is a way for cats to mark their territory. This leaves a visual scratch mark and an olfactory signature, but these must be frequently renewed to remain good markers.

ance, the tree is a territorial marker, readily visible to other cats that might venture through. In the process of scratching trees, a cat rubs secretions from glands in the front feet onto the tree trunk. Thus the scratched trunk gains an olfactory signature that can be recognized by other cats and that lets visitors know the territory is occupied. A territorial marker must be renewed if it is going to continue to communicate that the territory is occupied, so the feline territory owner is attracted back to the same tree to restore both the visual and chemical marks.

Scratching, whether on a tree, scratching post, or corner of a chair, also has the function of conditioning the claws. The claws are not sharpened as a knife blade would be sharpened,

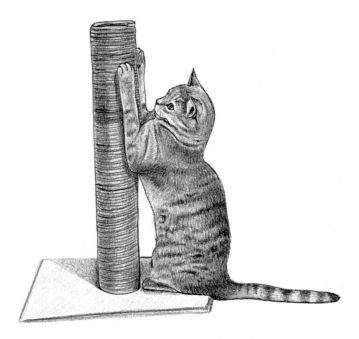

In the home most cats must have some sort of scratching "tree" as a territorial marker. The goal is to get them started on a tree substitute, a scratching post, from the beginning.

but frayed, worn outer claws are periodically pulled off by scratching, thus exposing new, sharp claws beneath. These removed worn claws can be seen at the base of a scratching post. Cats can also remove the frayed outer claws with their teeth; this is how they handle the claws of the back feet. Scratching is a natural, normal behavior and something for which we need to find an acceptable outlet.

Even inside the home, cats have a strong, innate tendency to establish at least one scratching-related territorial mark. If we are not careful, this will be the corner of a chair or couch that sticks out into a room and, to the cat, would be visible to strange cats walking through, which is what a marker is for. As soon as a cat starts scratching a particular object, it has kind of committed itself, and it tends to persist in scratching that object, coming back to it again and again.

When bringing a new kitten home, be thinking about the scratching behavior as much as the litter box. You should not wait until the cat is fully grown, and capable of serious damage, before training it to scratch on a particular object. In Chapter 2 on bringing home your new cat, we recommended also bringing home the scratching post the kitten is using. This post will be a natural one for your kitten to stay with in its new home. Place the post prominently in an area the kitten frequents, at least initially. Once the kitten is using the scratching post it can be gradually moved to a less conspicuous location.

When looking for a new scratching post, select one with a covering that allows for some nice long scratching. For a kitten it is useful to position the scratching post horizontally to make it easy for the kitten to develop an attachment to it. It also makes sense to demonstrate scratching by rubbing the kitten's front feet on the post. The kitten will not get your point about scratching, but by rubbing the kitten's feet on the post you are depositing some odors from the glands in the feet, and this should draw the kitten to the post.

If some scratching occurs on a piece of furniture, the scratched area should be covered immediately with a sheet of plastic to prevent further scratching and should be kept covered until the cat is regularly using the scratching post. You could place the post in front of the scratched furniture, or, if possible, temporarily move the furniture to another location.

Because cats tend to scratch just after awakening, they often develop a propensity for scratching objects near their sleeping areas. Therefore, it may be helpful to place scratching posts in those areas.

A good size for a scratching board is 6 to 8 inches in width by 12 to 16 inches in length. The height should be adjusted as the cat grows. The best height once the cat is grown is about 12 inches off the floor so that the cat may comfortably rest on its back feet while scratching. Gaining in popularity are scratching boards made of corrugated cardboard. The cardboard scratcher may be placed on the floor or attached to a vertical surface. When it comes time to replace a cardboard scratcher it would be wise to be sprinkle pieces of cardboard with the cat's foot odor from the old scratcher onto the new one. The material on a scratching post should be something a cat likes. Most commercial posts are covered with carpet, which actually is too durable. As a covering becomes worn out and stringy, the cat likes it better. Posts that are made of soft wood, such as pine, cedar, or redwood, are good choices, especially if roughened up with a wire brush.

You might be surprised to learn that there are differences between the breeds with regard to scratching up the furniture. The most likely to be problem scratchers are the Bengal, followed by the Abyssinian and Siamese. The least likely are the Persian, the hairless Sphynx, and the Cornish Rex.

Aggressive behavior

Episodes of aggressive behavior in cats generally are considered less problematic than litter box issues, urine marking in the home, or tearing up furniture. We mostly seem to know if a cat can be testy or likely to scratch us if picked up. The other problems mentioned cannot be handled by just ignoring them. Perhaps the biggest issue with a cat that tends toward aggression is that we often want to have an affection-loving cat—maybe like our last cat—but the cat's aggressive nature does not allow this. If having an affectionate cat is important to you, give some thought to getting a male, as well as a breed known for being nonaggressive, such as the Ragdoll, Burmese, or Maine Coon, as opposed to the Bengal or Abyssinian. The most aggressive cats tend to be the least affectionate.

One area in which early experience makes a big difference is in preventing aggression toward children. Young children especially can be perceived by cats as quite different from adults, and a cat may struggle or behave aggressively when a child tries to hold it, whereas with adults the same cat could be absolutely nonaggressive. Here is where front-loading the kitten with exposure and handling by children from the first day can pay off. If your family is expecting a child but none is present, borrow a relative's child frequently for kitten handling sessions and give the child a reward, such as M&Ms, for being really gentle; we suggest one M&M per minute of gentle handling.

• • •

Many problems can be avoided by investing time in shaping your kitten's behavior. Another approach is to select a breed or gender that is less prone to engage in these behaviors. In Chapter 3 we discussed gender differences with regard to some of these behavioral concerns, and breed differences are revealed in Chapter 6 and represented in the profiles in Chapter 7 for all of the problem behaviors discussed in this chapter. In addition, several books listed in the annotated bibliography offer very useful advice, and keep in mind that behavioral specialists can be consulted for serious problems.

Chapter 5

Historical background of cats

Before we delve into breed-specific behavioral characteristics in the next two chapters, it is useful to review the intriguing historical background of cat breeds and breed types. Particularly interesting is that some common breeds date way back in history to ancient Persia and Siam, while others stem from the efforts of breeders in the 1950s and 1960s.

But first we look just at the domestication of the cat, which began roughly 10,000 to 11,000 years ago, when humans stopped hunting and gathering and adopted a more agricultural lifestyle. As settled humans learned to grow grains, and grains became a dietary staple, the small wild cats hanging around the farms were beneficial for the control of rodents, who savored the same dietary staple as humans. From about this time on, cats tied their evolutionary fate to human settlements and, you might say, vice versa. Many of these cats eventually became household pets, and the process of domestication began.

Recent genetic research reveals that domestic cats, as we know them, stem from a single domestication event in the Near East. The early domesticated cats, being attached to their humans, spread to virtually all parts of Asia and Europe along trade routes between ancient civilizations. Eventually, genetically distinguishable groups of cat types arose in Asia, East Africa, the Mediterranean Basin, and Western Europe. The cats that were introduced to North America as part of the settlers' possessions were those closely linked to the Western European cats.

An interesting aspect of cat domestication is that as global migration continued, many developing breeds remained quite similar to their felid ancestors in form and function. Compared with the dog and other common domesticated animals, the modern cat is not as fully domesticated, or altered, genetically. Cats of many breeds that become feral, living on their own, are self-sufficient with hunting skills, and in many villages around the world cats continue with the work of controlling rodent pests.

When we read about the early development of dog breeds, we discover that the overwhelming emphasis has been on breeding working companions. Through selective breeding for "hardwired" working behavioral roles, dog breeds have become specialized in body form and behavior for such tasks as herding sheep, pointing to and retrieving game birds, chasing foxes, and protecting the property from intruders. For early domestic cats, the working role of hunting down rodent pests came naturally, and this was the only job that was ever expected. Over time, of course, people got rid of open grain storage and rodent pests pretty much became a thing of the past. The valued working role of catching rodent pests shows up now in the cat bringing home the rat and leaving it on the doorstep.

At the time that feline pest control on farms became less important, people began to realize that by selective breeding they could change body style and size, hair coat, and many aspects of behavior. Much selective breeding has been for a sense of grace and beauty, at least in the eyes of the human beholder.

Various body styles have become associated with cats in certain parts of the world. Subsets of cats that had similar body styles, and that had undergone intensive selection for maintaining those signature body styles, became the ancestral purebred or pedigree cats. The ancestral purebreds made up the first group of breeds recognized by the cat fancy associations. The development of new body styles has been rather rapid recently because the selection has occurred with just a single gene, rather than with multiple genes, which is a more complex process.

The oldest identifiable cat breed is the Persian, with the stocky body and long hair giving the breed its graceful look. Apparently the early breeders thought a stub-nosed (brachycephalic) head type was attractive and concentrated on the signature look. Obviously here is a family cat that couldn't help much with the rodent pest control if it wanted. As the name implies, the Persian originated in ancient Persia (now Iran).

In another part of the ancient world, Siam (now Thailand), breeders went in the opposite direction of the Persian breeders and selected for a long, sleek, lithe cat with large pointed ears, almond-shaped blue eyes, and a wedged-shaped (doliocephalic) head. Both the Siamese and Persian are very old identifiable breeds, and they exemplify the range of body types that go way back in feline history.

The body style characteristics of the Persian and Siamese breeds are paired up with major differences in behavior. Persians are the lowest ranking of all breeds we looked at in activity level, playfulness, vocalization, furniture scratching, and predatory behavior. In contrast, the Siamese is the highest ranking of all breeds in vocalization and among the highest ranking in activity level, playfulness, and furniture scratching. The Siamese is also above average in going after songbirds and certainly retains its rodent pest control predisposition. If need be, the Siamese could still be counted upon to protect the grain storage.

As imaginations grew in cat breeding circles, selective breeding for body style produced large cats that thrived in cold winters, such as the tailless Manx, the Norwegian Forest Cat, and the Maine Coon, the latter being the largest of all cats, and larger than some dogs. Other breeders were determined to get a hairless cat, resulting in the Sphynx.

Breed development continues today, with some breeds quickly becoming very popular. One is the Ragdoll, out of Southern California in the 1960s, and known for its affectionate nature and very low level of aggression toward other cats or people—a cat you can push across the floor with a slipper, like a ragdoll. The modern contrast to the Ragdoll, and also from Southern California in the 1960s, is the very active, beautifully styled Bengal, the opposite of the Ragdoll in behavior, with aggressive tendencies toward other cats and people, with little interest in affection, and mostly wanting to make an urban forest out of the furniture in your home. Although this breed got its wildcat boost from the Asian Leopard Cat, the founders of the breed seemed to think reference to the Bengal tiger was more romantic.

The intent of this chapter is to briefly discuss the interesting historical background of modern-day cats—from ancient, slow-moving Persia and Siam to much less ancient, and much less patient, Southern California. Over time, cat fanciers have proven to be about as diverse in envisioning their ideal cat as dog fanciers have in envisioning their ideal dog. In Chapter 7, where we discuss individual breeds, you will see that each has a particular developmental story.

Chapter 6

Understanding behavioral characteristics of cats

When people select a dog, the questions asked about behavior invariably reflect what is known, or assumed, about breed differences, even if the intent is to get a dog from a shelter. We know that behavioral differences among dog breeds usually reflect some utilitarian role in the breed's background such as herding sheep, retrieving game for hunters, and chasing rats out of burrows.

When it comes to cats, most people are not as focused on behavior, perhaps because they are not aware of the real behavioral differences that exist among the various breeds of cats. We know that a Collie is not nearly as active as a Jack Russell Terrier, and that a Golden Retriever is more affectionate than a Husky, but we may not know the extent to which an Abyssinian is more aggressive than a Burmese, or the degree to which the Manx is less affectionate than the Ragdoll. Interestingly, the behavioral differences among cat breeds seem to be the result of an intentional focus on breeding for certain companionable behaviors, as well as looks and body style.

In this chapter we focus on twelve behavioral characteristics of cats to see how fifteen of the most commonly recognized breeds, as well as the generic domestic shorthair (DSH) and domestic longhair (DLH), differ. The graph for each behavior trait ranks the breeds and shows the degree to which breeds differ in that behavior. The underlying assumption is that behavior differences, like body style, are largely genetically based.

We can imagine the day, when more advances have been made in behavioral genetics, that we could do a DNA analysis of a kitten of unknown parentage and get a preview of the behaviors that would likely emerge as the kitten becomes an adult. This brings us to the point of discussing how the data on the behavioral traits were obtained. Vague descriptions such as "good natured," "self-confident," "versatile," "cute," "dignified," and "wonderful companion" are not very useful when you want specific information, such as whether a breed has a tendency to be affectionate, good at litter box use, not easily provoked to urine marking, or not likely to be aggressive toward people.

Reflecting the statistical analyses that were used to analyze our raw data, as explained below, the behavioral characteristics vary in predictive value. That is, a trait with a high predictive value (represented by the statistical notation "F value") is better at distinguishing between breeds than a trait with a much lower predictive value. The following twelve traits are listed in decreasing order of predictive value.

Traits with the highest predictive value

Vocalization	(F value = 22.0)
Activity level	(F value = 18.6)
Predation on songbirds	(F value = 18.2)

Traits with moderate predictive value

Aggression toward family members   (F value = 8.8)
Affection toward family members   (F value = 8.6)
Playfulness   (F value = 7.8)
Aggression toward other cats   (F value = 7.4)
Litter box use   (F value = 6.9)
Furniture scratching   (F value = 6.3)
Urine marking in the home   (F value = 5.7)

Traits with the lowest predictive value

Friendliness toward visitors   (F value = 4.3)
Fearfulness of strangers   (F value = 3.4)

How the rankings were obtained

In the behavioral traits covered here, breeds are ranked on a scale of one to ten, with one designating the lowest rank and ten the highest rank. Whether a rank of one or ten is more desirable depends on the behavior and the preferences of the person using the rankings. For example, almost everyone would want a kitten to rank tops in litter box use and low in urine marking tendency. But when it comes to activity level, some people prefer an inactive cat that mostly lies around, while others want an active cat that provides a bit of entertainment.

In addition to breed differences, gender also plays a role in behavior. In Chapter 3 we discussed differences between neutered males and spayed females with regard to these same twelve behavior traits, and you will want to consider these differences when making your breed selection.

The graphs in this chapter represent the cumulative rankings of eighty veterinarians specializing in feline practice—both male and female feline practitioners, randomly chosen to represent eastern, central, and western areas of the United

States—whom we consider to be unbiased authorities on breed differences in cats. If anyone should have an overall understanding of differences between the various cat breeds and between the sexes, it is these authorities.

Each practitioner was interviewed for twenty to thirty minutes, during which time the practitioner was given a brief description of each of the twelve behavior traits. The practitioner was first asked to compare neutered male and spayed female cats without reference to breed, and then to rank a list of seven breeds (five purebreds, chosen randomly from the master list of fifteen purebreds, plus the DSH and DLH). A computer program then assembled the individual rankings from all authorities, for all breeds, and for all twelve behavior traits, and calculated an average score for each breed, plus the DSH and DLH. The scores obtained are what statisticians refer to as the least squares mean. This mean was then adjusted to fall in the range of one to ten, with one the lowest ranking and ten the highest ranking.

These graphs depict relative ranks, not absolute scores. Thus, for the trait of affection, a score of ten does not mean perfectly affectionate and a score of one does not mean a complete lack of affection. A low-ranking score on litter box use does not mean an absence of litter box habits, nor does having the highest ranking on litter box use indicate infallibility in this regard. The graphs specify that there is a range in the trait among breeds, as experienced by caregivers and conveyed to their feline veterinarians. Thus, selecting a breed that ranks high in affection makes sense if what you want is a very affectionate cat that loves to be held. But all breeds have the potential to be affectionate, even if they are in the lowest ranks. The graphs portray relative tendencies, not absolute differences. And, it is very important to note that there is individual variability within each breed with regard to each characteristic.

How to evaluate the rankings

As mentioned, the rankings of the twelve traits are averages expressed as least squares means adjusted to rank the breeds from one to ten, with ten being the highest ranking. In terms of statistical differences, for any behavioral trait, the three highest ranking breeds are usually different than the three lowest ranking breeds. Those in the middle will not differ much from one another, but could well differ from the highest and/or lowest ranked breeds. The lengths of the bars in the graphs tell you a lot. When a bar is considerably longer or shorter than other bars, it is a clear sign of a statistically significant difference.

Using the graphs in this chapter, together with the graphs in Chapter 7, allows you to search for your ideal cat. If you are going to either select or rule out a breed based on a particular trait, the trait should have a high, or at least moderate, predictive value. It follows that the environment will have more of an effect on the traits that do not distinguish themselves as well among breeds. As you will see in Chapter 7, some behavioral traits go together. The affectionate breeds are usually the least aggressive, for instance.

Finally, it is important to re-emphasize that there are behavioral differences among individual cats within a given breed. These differences are a result of particular blood lines, the behavior of the mother and father, and the environment of the breeder in shaping the early experience. The setting in which you place a kitten—your home—will also affect behavior.

Breed differences in the behavioral characteristics

For each behavioral characteristic a question was presented to the authorities. The authorities were asked to compare males with females and to then rank the seven breeds assigned to them.

Vocalization
Predictive value: highest

Many companion cats are so quiet you may hardly know they are around. But then there are the cats that, according to caregivers, seem to be incessant "talkers."

Most people know that the Siamese are the most outspoken of cat breeds. As a reflection of this common knowledge, the trait of vocalization turned out to have the highest predictive value of all traits. This means that if you are using the information in this book to help you select a kitten to be the least, or the most, vocal as an adult, your selection should be accurate.

So, let's say you want a vocal cat, but you like the looks and other behavior traits of a Tonkinese. You can bet that cats of this breed will be pretty vocal—they let you know they are around—but not as noisy as the Siamese. The quietest breeds are the Persian, Maine Coon, and Ragdoll.

The following statement was presented to the ranking authorities: *"Some cats, as adults, appear to be naturally more talkative than others with regard to frequency and intensity of vocalizations. While some cat caregivers may encourage or discourage this behavior, there may be gender as well as breed differences in this regard."* The authorities were asked to first compare males with females without regard to breed and then to rank the seven breeds assigned to them without regard to gender.

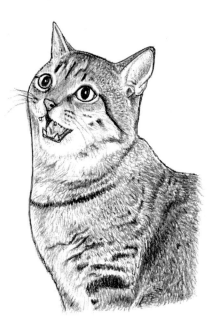

Vocalization

Lowest ranked: Persian
Highest ranked: Siamese

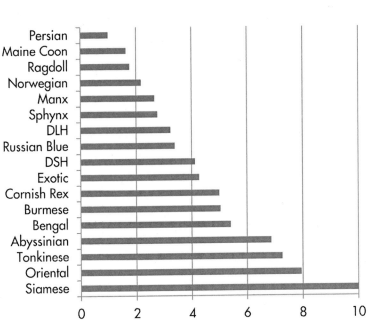

Ranking of the breeds from least to most likely to be vocal.

Activity level
Predictive value: high

General activity refers to how much a cat moves about without being stimulated, as well as its tendency to be activated by a stimulus, such as someone dragging a lamp cord across the floor. This characteristic is one on which prospective cat adopters are going to differ with regard to what they find desirable. Some adopters will prefer a high level of activity and love seeing the cat race across the yard, while others are just as happy with an inactive cat. Most folks will be happy with a moderate degree of moving about.

The Bengal and Abyssinian stand out as the most active breeds. These are the cats that like to make a three-dimensional forest out of our bookshelves and mantels when not racing across the floor. The least active breed is the Persian, which you can almost guess just by looking at its body type. The Ragdoll also scores low in activity level, probably taking to hanging around and being petted rather than exploring the environment. The DSH and the DLH rank at the moderate level.

Because the predictive value of this trait is high, you will be more successful in predicting a kitten's activity level as an adult than you would be predicting a kitten's level of fearfulness as an adult, which is a trait with a low predictive value. Traits with the highest predictive value are less influenced by environment and training than those with a lower predictive value.

The following statement was presented to the ranking authorities: *"Some cats appear to be naturally more active—they move about more, or are more restless than others—and there may be gender as well as breed differences in this regard."* The authorities were asked to first compare males with females without regard to breed and then to rank the seven breeds assigned to them without regard to gender.

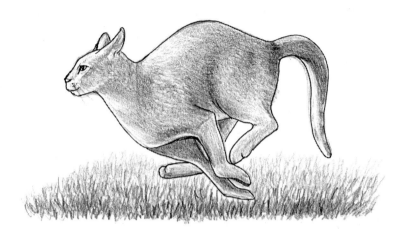

Activity level

Lowest ranked: Persian • Highest ranked: Bengal

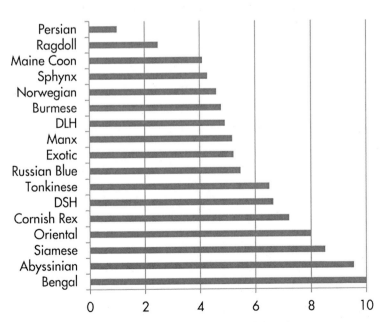

Ranking of the breeds from least to most likely to be active.

Predation on songbirds
Predictive value: high

It can be heartbreaking for some of us to see a young fledgling taken, even though the cat is simply being a "normal cat." Of course this problem is nonexistent if the cat is never allowed outside. But this may not be feasible in some instances.

The breeds highest in songbird predation are those that are most active and wild in behavior, the Bengal and Abyssinian. The DSH and DLH also rank rather high. Those with the lowest tendency to prey on songbirds are the relatively inactive Persian and the Sphynx. The Ragdoll, followed by the Cornish Rex, rank relatively low in this trait. Given the high predictive value of this trait, you should be reliable in selecting a breed of kitten from the low end if you do not want the cat to be a predator and it will have access to the outdoors.

The following statement was presented to the ranking authorities: *"For cats that have access to the outdoors, some, as adults, appear to have a stronger tendency to prey on songbirds than others, and there may be gender as well as breed differences in this regard."* The authorities were asked to first compare males with females without regard to breed and then to rank the seven breeds assigned to them without regard to gender.

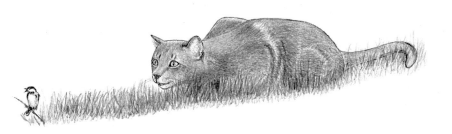

Predation on songbirds

Lowest ranked: Persian • Highest ranked: Domestic shorthair

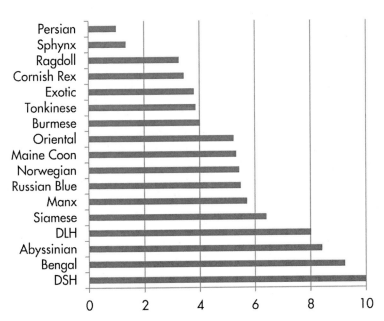

Ranking of the breeds from least to most likely to prey on songbirds.

Aggression toward family members
Predictive value: moderate

Here is a behavior that can be directed toward just one or several family members; the behavior may be variable, and the cat is likely to be aggressive at some times but not at other times. We do not necessarily mean outright biting or scratching, but threatening by means of posture or growling. The aggression may range from rather mild to very noticeable.

Especially if you have young children, you may want to choose a breed with a very low tendency for aggression. According to our authorities, the Ragdoll is clearly the least aggressive; just look at the graph and the relative length of the bar. Also having a low tendency toward aggression are the Sphynx, Burmese, and Maine Coon.

Selecting a cat just for its awesome wild looks, such as the Bengal or the Abyssinian, can get you a more aggressive cat, which is fine if you know what you are getting, but which could spell trouble if you are not expecting this.

The following statement was presented to the ranking authorities: *"While we recognize that there may be experiences that influence aggression, some cats, as adults, appear to be naturally more aggressive toward human family members than others in terms of growling, scratching, and biting, and there may be gender and breed differences in this regard."* The authorities were asked to first compare males with females without regard to breed and then to rank the seven breeds assigned to them without regard to gender.

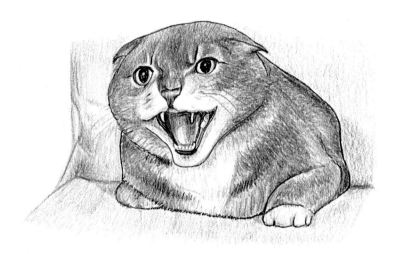

Aggression toward family members
Lowest ranked: Ragdoll • Highest ranked: Bengal

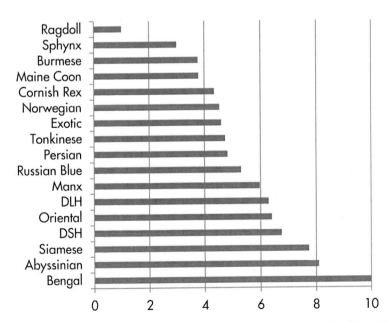

Ranking of the breeds from least to most likely to show aggression toward family members.

Affection toward family members
Predictive value: moderate

Probably what most of us notice more than anything else is how affectionate our cat is. Whether we are reading a book, curled up on the couch watching the latest feature of reality TV, or sharing our bed with the feline family member, assuring affection from our cat can mean a lot. In animal assisted therapy, nonjudgmental affection represents the therapeutic mission of the cat. The Ragdoll, the breed highest ranked on this trait, is well known for being affectionate. The DSH and the Burmese are the next most affectionate.

But affection does not top everyone's priority list. Some caregivers enjoy just watching a cat with striking looks, such as the much less affectionate Bengal, moving about the home. Affection would be nice, but cats can be appreciated in their own right. One could say the same for the low-ranking tailless Manx. These cats have a following perhaps based on their distinctive looks. An interesting question is how the hairless Sphynx, which might not look like it would be very affectionate, and definitely feels different to the touch, ranks. According to our authorities, the Sphynx ranks in the middle.

The following statement was presented to the ranking authorities: *"While we recognize that there may be experiences that influence affection, some cats, as adults, appear to be naturally more affectionate toward family members than others, and there may be gender as well as breed differences in this regard."* The authorities were asked to first compare males with females without regard to breed and then to rank the seven breeds assigned to them without regard to gender.

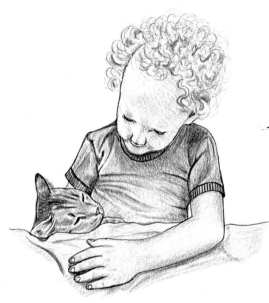

Affection toward family members

Lowest ranked: Bengal
Highest ranked: Ragdoll

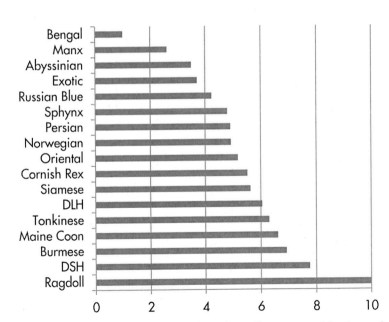

Ranking of the breeds from least to most likely to show affection toward family members.

Playfulness
Predictive value: moderate

We all expect kittens to play a lot. But if cats were more like us, they would outgrow much of their playfulness. As it turns out, in the development of some breeds we have emphasized playfulness in the cats as adults, while in others we have selected for a less playful predisposition.

Some people love playfulness in their adult cat and encourage it by providing toys and joining in the play. Clearly the most playful is the Abyssinian, also one of the most active breeds. Not far behind are the DSH and the Bengal. Ranking very low in playfulness is the Persian, which is the least active breed. Also on the non-playful side are the Sphynx and the Norwegian Forest Cat, which also rank low in activity.

The following statement was presented to the ranking authorities: *"Some cats may appear to be naturally more playful, as adults, than others, with human family members or with other cats, and there may be gender as well as breed differences in this regard."* The authorities were asked to first compare males with females without regard to breed and then to rank the seven breeds assigned to them without regard to gender.

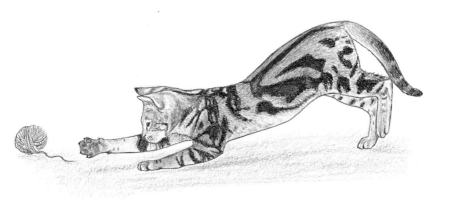

Playfulness
Lowest ranked: Persian • Highest ranked: Abyssinian

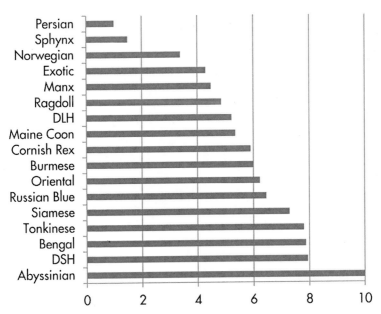

Ranking of the breeds from least to most likely to be playful.

Aggression toward other cats
Predictive value: moderate

In a multi-cat household, a cat that generally gets along well with other cats is less trouble than one that is habitually threatening others. Aggression toward other cats is not infrequent in multi-cat homes and often just reflects the asocial predisposition of the feline ancestors that lived a solitary lifestyle in Africa and had a tendency to fend off strangers. In domestic cats we have selected for some breeds to be more socially accepting of other cats in the household.

If you have already looked at the breed graphs in Chapter 7, you will not be surprised to find that the Ragdoll is the least aggressive toward other cats. The Cornish Rex, Burmese, and Sphynx also rank at the low end, but not nearly as low as the Ragdoll. The rather wild Bengal ranks the highest in aggression toward other cats, and not far behind are the Siamese and Abyssinian. The DSH, Oriental, and DLH also rank at the high end.

The following statement was presented to the ranking authorities: *"Some cats seem to be naturally more aggressive toward other cats, with a tendency to readily growl or start fights, while others may be friendlier toward other cats in the same house, and there may be gender as well as breed differences in this regard."* The authorities were asked to first compare males with females without regard to breed and then to rank the seven breeds assigned to them without regard to gender.

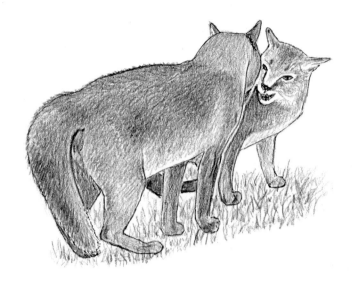

Aggression toward other cats
Lowest ranked: Ragdoll • Highest ranked: Bengal

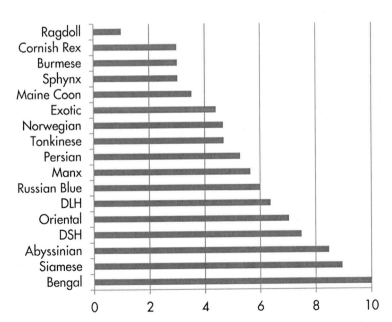

Ranking of the breeds from least to most likely to show aggression toward other cats.

Litter box use
Predictive value: moderate

Because cats tend to have fastidious sanitary behavior, they can make an ideal, low-maintenance, housemate with no walks required for elimination; just clean the soiled litter twice a day. Here is a behavior—digging a hole and burying feces and urine—that works well not only in nature but also in our homes. But, beware, not all cats are the same in this regard. According to our authorities, who hear about litter box issues when they arise, there are real differences among breeds.

The impressive thing about the litter box use graph is the rather tight grouping of breeds, with the exception of the Persian, which clearly ranks low. This breed, arguably the oldest and bred over centuries for inactivity, seems to have carried with it some inactivity with regard to litter box use.

The following statement was presented to the ranking authorities: *"While we recognize that there may be management factors that affect litter box use, some cats naturally seem to take to using a litter box, and to maintaining this sanitary behavior, more than do other cats, and there may be gender as well as breed differences in this regard."* The authorities were asked to first compare males with females without regard to breed and then to rank the seven breeds assigned to them without regard to gender.

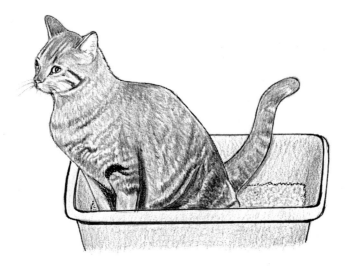

Litter box use

Lowest ranked: Persian • Highest ranked: Domestic shorthair

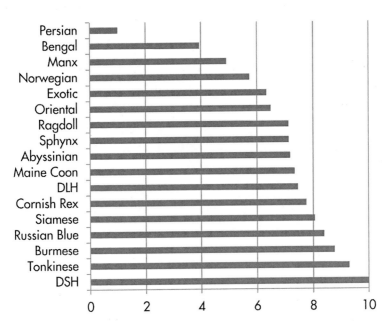

Ranking of the breeds from least to most likely to use a litter box consistently.

Furniture scratching
Predictive value: moderate

Other than urine marking, probably no behavior makes a cat less welcome in our homes than tearing up the furniture by clawing or scratching. To cats, they are just marking their territory so other cats wandering through can see and smell that Benny the Bengal lives here. After all, this is what cats do in nature with trees in their territory. Once cats begin to scratch an object, they stay with that object. In nature this means that the same tree is repeatedly scratched, maintaining the scratched appearance as well as the scent from the foot glands. The same holds with the territory marker that is in the living room. And that's why the corners of the couch or chairs get torn to shreds.

The breed that is tops in furniture scratching is also the most active, and if you will, wild-like—the Bengal. Not too far behind are the Siamese and Abyssinian. The least likely to engage in furniture scratching is the rather inactive Persian, followed by the hairless Sphynx and the Cornish Rex.

The following statement was presented to the ranking authorities: *"Even with access to an appropriate scratching object, such as a scratching post, some cats may have a stronger tendency than others to scratch household furniture, and there may be gender as well as breed differences in this regard."* The authorities were asked to first compare males with females without regard to breed and then to rank the seven breeds assigned to them without regard to gender.

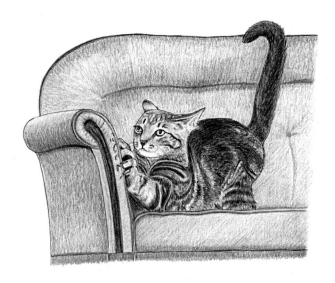

Furniture scratching

Lowest ranked: Persian • Highest ranked: Bengal

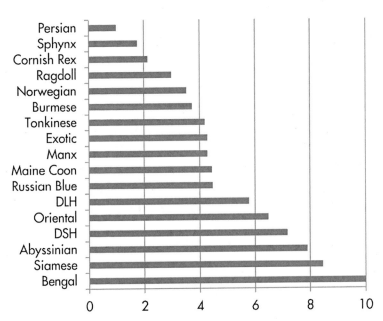

Ranking of the breeds from least to most likely to scratch furniture.

Urine marking in the home
Predictive value: moderate

Here is a behavior that virtually all cat caregivers want to avoid. This is a natural, innate behavior for the ancestral cat, one of a number of forms of territory marking. As stated in earlier chapters, several factors influence whether or not a cat will urine mark in the home, but the main factor is gender. Males are much more likely than females to urine mark. Urine marking behavior in males is highly dependent on the sex hormone, testosterone. Cats are seasonally reproductive, and testosterone levels in males vary by season. During the off season, urine marking is not so prevalent. Most neutered males do not urine mark, but enough of them do that this behavior is the most common problem behavior for which medical treatment is sought.

DSH cats are ranked highest in urine marking, with the Bengal, DLH, and Siamese not far behind. The least likely to urine mark is the Sphynx. (We wonder if being hairless in some way is incompatible with urine spraying; it would certainly look embarrassing.) The Cornish Rex and Ragdoll also rank low in urine marking.

The following statement was presented to the ranking authorities: *"While we recognize that there are environmental factors that may lead to urine marking in the home, some cats are more likely than others to engage in this behavior, and there may be gender as well as breed differences in this regard."* The authorities were asked to first compare males with females without regard to breed and then to rank the seven breeds assigned to them without regard to gender.

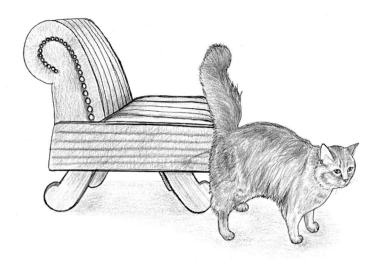

Urine marking in the home

Lowest ranked: Sphynx • Highest ranked: Domestic shorthair

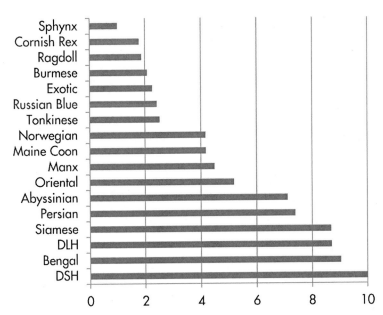

Ranking of the breeds from least to most likely to urine mark in the home.

Friendliness toward visitors
Predictive value: low

When people come over to visit and your cat just takes to them, showing its affection by rubbing against them and asking to be petted, your visitors can feel more welcome. In fact, visitors can easily take this as validation that they are trusted by animals and, therefore, seen as a good person. A family cat that is social toward visitors, or even strangers, is usually favored.

Considering the low predictability of this trait we can assume, at least, that the high-ranking Ragdoll and Maine Coon kittens will grow up to be welcoming of guests, as long as experiences with visitors are positive, and that the low-ranking Persian, Sphynx, and Exotic kittens, as adults, are least likely to be social. The Persian's tendency to be the least social fits with its tendency to be fearful of strangers as well.

The following statement was presented to the ranking authorities: *"While we recognize that there are factors that may alter the degree to which a cat is socially outgoing, some cats appear to be naturally more friendly than others with relative strangers, and there may be gender as well as breed differences in this regard."* The authorities were asked to first compare males with females without regard to breed and then to rank the seven breeds assigned to them without regard to gender.

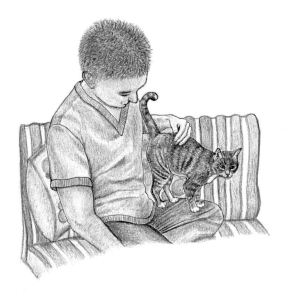

Friendliness toward visitors

Lowest ranked: Persian • Highest ranked: Ragdoll

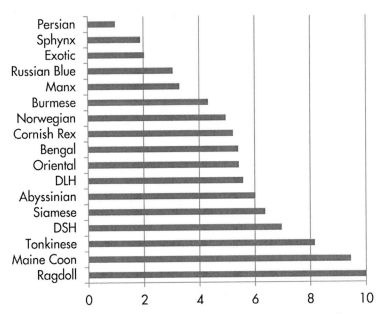

Ranking of the breeds from least to most likely to be friendly to visitors.

Fearfulness of strangers
Predictive value: lowest

When friends come to visit you, your cat can be outgoing and social, or indifferent, or fearful and hide. For the most part, we like our cats to be welcoming with visitors, but if that is too much to ask, at least not fearful and hiding.

Clearly, the most fearful cat is the Persian; one could say, they just like a calm home—no visitors to upset the routine, thank you.

The least fearful, by quite a margin, is the Ragdoll; you could say they consider visitors fun—the more to pet and hold you. The Maine Coon and Tonkinese are also on the least fearful side. All of this said, this trait has the least predictive value of all. In other words, selecting a breed on the basis of not being fearful, is less reliable than selecting a breed on the basis of other traits. Keep in mind that the more early experience a kitten has in being introduced to visitors, the less fearful they will be as adults. The main takeaway message is that the Persian is at one end of the scale and the Ragdoll at the other.

The following statement was presented to the ranking authorities: *"While we recognize that there are factors that may alter the degree to which a cat is fearful, some cats, as adults, appear to be naturally more fearful, standoffish, or withdrawn than others with regard to people visiting the home, and there may be gender as well as breed differences in this regard."* The authorities were asked to first compare males with females without regard to breed and then to rank the seven breeds assigned to them without regard to gender.

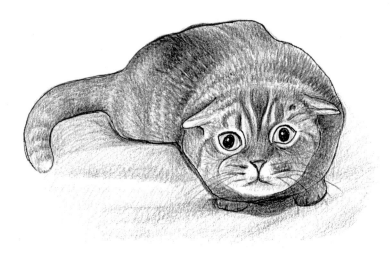

Fearfulness of strangers

Lowest ranked: Ragdoll • Highest ranked: Persian

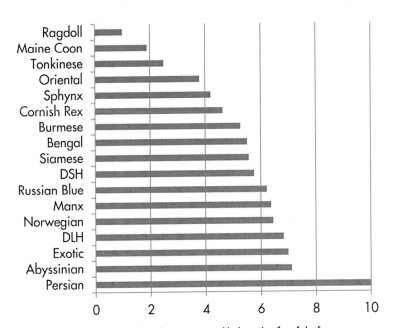

Ranking of the breeds from least to most likely to be fearful of strangers.

• • •

The twelve graphs in this chapter provide a fairly accurate over-all view of the behavioral differences among breeds. There may be some surprises here, even for those who have a lot of experience with cats. Remember that these graphs do not reflect the opinions of the authors but instead represent the statistical consensus of eighty feline authorities. And an important point to keep in mind is that superimposed on the breed differences are individual differences stemming from environmental factors and genetic variability within a breed.

Combining the data on each behavioral trait for the different breeds is the feature of the next chapter.

Chapter 7

Behavioral profiles of cat breeds

The collection of behavioral profiles that follow is a central feature of this book. It is essential to keep in mind what these profiles mean and what they do and do not tell you. The graphs represent not the authors' opinions but the results of interviewing eighty small-animal veterinarians specializing in feline medicine. These authorities were divided between men and women from the eastern, central, and western parts of the United States. Each was asked to rank a list of seven breeds on each of the twelve behavioral traits, discussed in Chapter 6. Of these seven breeds to rank, five were breeds of cats chosen at random from the master list of fifteen purebreds, plus the generic domestic shorthair (DSH) and domestic longhair (DLH). Sometimes the term domestic medium hair (DMH) is used by some, but this is uncommon and authorities were not asked to rank the DMH cat.

These authorities were not allowed to include cat breeds of their own choosing, so the evaluations should be relatively free of personal biases. A computer program was designed to process the eighty sets of rankings to create a series of rankings for all fifteen purebreds plus the DSH and DLH. These rankings were then used to generate a behavioral profile graph for each breed or breed type.

How to use the behavioral profiles

You will probably enjoy thumbing through the profiles to look at some of the breeds with which you are already familiar, and you may want to compare how closely the behavioral profiles match your experience with individual cats. Keep in mind that there is variation among individual cats within a breed and that these profiles represent a statistical consensus of eighty feline authorities, who have seen many cats from each purebred breed, as well as the DSH and DLH. Your recollections about the behavior of a particular cat of a certain breed thus will not necessarily match the profile presented here. Likewise, if you are an authority yourself on one or more cat breeds and feel that some of the profiles are out of line with your own experience, remember that these rankings are not the opinions of the authors but a statistical consensus of authorities.

While the breed profiles approximate the relative differences between breeds, do not take the graphs too literally. The difference between a breed ranking third on a trait versus one ranking fourth or fifth is probably insignificant. You can, however, probably count on the differences in breeds that rank at the lowest end of a scale to be quite different from the breeds that rank at the higher end. If having a cat that is highly affectionate is a top priority, look at breeds ranking in the top one-third of the affection scale.

Included in the breed profiles are references to body size, hair coat, and medical problems that seem most prominent for that breed and presumably reflect a genetic predisposition.

Another factor, just as important in determining a cat's adult behavior, is the specific genetic contribution made to an animal by its mother and father. If the behavior of the mother and father seem to match the behavioral profile presented here, there is a very good chance that the kitten you choose will as an adult behave along the same lines predicted.

Throughout your selection process, if a breeder expresses opinions about a breed that differ from the profile presented here, recall that you are hearing that one person's opinion. In fact, we suspect that some breeders will be unhappy with various rankings. No breeder is likely to be delighted that his or her breed is ranked high on urine marking or aggressive tendencies. However, the way the breeds are ranked is similar to how a class of students taking an exam is ranked. Not all students can get the top score; there is a student with the highest score and one with the lowest. If you're looking for the best breeds with regard to a particular trait, look at those that are top ranked. But if a trait is not of particular importance to you, the ranking may not make any difference. Our philosophy is that different breeds of cats are suited for different environments, and that for each breed there is a particular home or environment for which it is quite suitable.

The fifteen purebred breeds are discussed in alphabetical order, followed by the DSH and DLH.

Abyssinian

To quote one authority, "Living with an Abyssinian is like living with a monkey." This is a reference to the Abyssinian's well-known reputation for being among the most active of cat breeds, and also to its having been bred to retain its somewhat wild looks. The reputation for a high activity level is verified by the breed profile graph, with its activity level bar near the very top. You can see why they are often likened to monkeys.

Abyssinians can dictate your home decorating style. These cats operate in three-dimensional space, not surface area. Forget putting up knickknack shelves with family glass heirlooms and instead only display items that can withstand a bounce on the floor. Aficionados of this breed not only referred to the high level of activity but also the lightning-fast manner that characterizes the Abyssinian's movement about its environment. Fans of this breed emphasize that it is necessary to provide a vertical structure or a cat post or two for the Aby to enjoy.

The Abyssinian is one of the breeds named after the country in which it presumably lived prior to its introduction to Europe—in this case Abyssinia (now Ethiopia). While history has it that the breed was from Abyssinia and brought to England in the 1870s, more recent genetic tracing locates the Abyssinian's origin in Southeast Asia and around the Indian Ocean, without a specific country identified. Abyssinians are known for their long legs and modified wedge-shaped head. Their caregivers tend to like the rather wild look, but actually there are other breeds, particularly the Bengal, closer in genetic proximity to one of the wild cats.

As well as ranking at the top (alongside Bengals) for all-out activity level, the Abys are not great lap cats, although they are far from bottom ranking in affection, and you can expect to get in some warm petting. Aby caregivers undoubtedly

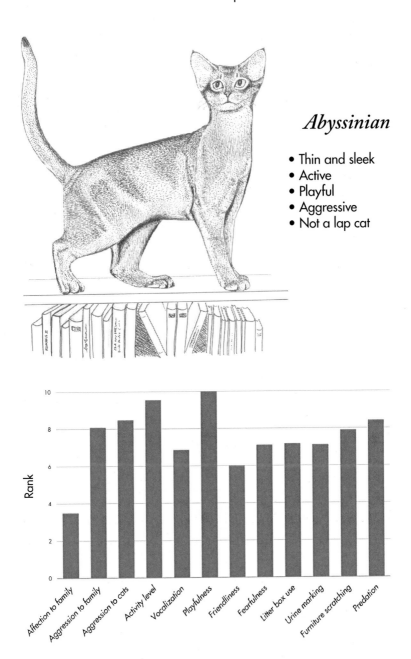

Abyssinian

- Thin and sleek
- Active
- Playful
- Aggressive
- Not a lap cat

Ranking of the Abyssinian on the twelve behavioral traits. The higher the ranking, the more likely the cat will exhibit this trait.

love the playfulness of this breed, which is tops. But be fore-warned—the Abys rank quite high in aggression toward both human and feline family members and therefore feel most at home being the only cat in the family.

Take note that the Abyssinian is in the top group in terms of tendency to engage in urine marking behavior. It is also top ranked in furniture scratching. Songbird predation, for those Abys that have access to the outdoors, is ranked at the top, again, something you might expect from such an active cat. Given the Aby's tendency toward urine marking, here is a breed in which selecting a female makes sense. On the other hand, selecting a male provides an edge with regard to more affection and less aggression.

Because they are of the shorthair variety, Abyssinians require little grooming beyond just regular petting. With regard to genetically related medical problems, a kidney disease referred to as renal amyloidosis has been reported, as have cardiomyopathy and some skin problems.

Bengal

Imagine a scene in which a miniature Asian leopard peers out from behind the vases, photographs, and plants on the mantel mounted above your fireplace. If this scene appeals to you, and you're not looking for this leopard cat to sit in your lap or insist on snuggling with you, then the Bengal may be for you. As a matter of fact, the Bengal is the cat for many, and it is one of the fastest growing breeds in popularity of recent years.

The Bengal is closely related to the Asian Leopard Cat, a wild cat that traces its ancestry to India, over to China, and down through the Malaysian peninsula. The most prominent feature of this breed is its hair coat and coloration. The fur is very dense, and the spots, or rather rosettes, and stripes on the Bengal were selected to closely mimic those of the leopard. Breeders wanted this cat to look different from all other domestic cats.

So how did this breed get started? Authorities attribute the origin of the Bengal to Jean Mill of Southern California who, in 1963, actually owned a wild female Asian Leopard Cat, similar to one she had spotted on a trip to the jungles of Southeast Asia. In those days Leopard Cats were sold in pet shops that specialized in selling exotic animals. Ms. Mill added a black male DSH to keep her wild Leopard Cat company. The offspring of the mating were sterile when bred together, but females of that first generation were bred again to DSH males to produce at least some fertile offspring. Further selective breeding with another male Leopard Cat, obtained from a zoo in India, brought out the very distinctive leopard-like colorations we are familiar with today. The intention of early breeders was to try to create a cat with the wild looks of a leopard and the calmer temperament of the domestic cat.

As initially developed, the Bengal was, by definition, a hybrid. Over time this designation will probably no longer hold, but due to its hybrid background the Bengal has not been accepted by the largest cat registry, the Cat Fanciers' Association (CFA). However, the International Cat Association and the American Cat Fanciers Association (ACFA) do register this breed.

While fanciers of the Bengal like to refer to this cat as being completely domesticated, a glance at the behavioral profile may give you some pause. It scores lowest on affection toward family members and the highest on aggression toward family members and aggression toward other cats. It also ranks highest on activity level. Even if some fanciers of this breed disagree with our authorities' rankings, it is generally acknowledged that Bengals are very active cats, and also very playful. You will want to protect your precious knickknacks from being knocked off the shelf by your Bengal dashing from "limb to limb" in its urban forest.

As you might expect from this description of the Bengal, the behavioral profile reflects activities that benefit cats in the wild, particularly the highest ranking for marking their territory by scratching (the corner of the couch substitutes nicely for a tree) and top ranking for spraying urine. And when it does get access to the outdoors, our data suggest that the Bengal is one of the breeds most likely to prey on songbirds.

The short hair coat of the Bengal needs relatively little upkeep. A weekly brushing could be nice, but don't struggle with the cat to get this done. After all, wild cats do well in nature with self-grooming. In fact the rather rough tongue surface with papillae does an excellent job of keeping the coat of short-haired cats in good shape.

While no specific disease vulnerabilities are apparent at this time, an interesting feature stemming from its Asian Leopard Cat ancestry is that the Bengal seems to have an actual immunity to feline leukemia virus, and it is often used in research studies on that disease.

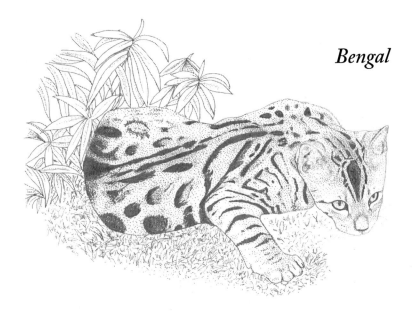

Bengal

Leopard-like beauty • Active • Aggressive • Not affectionate

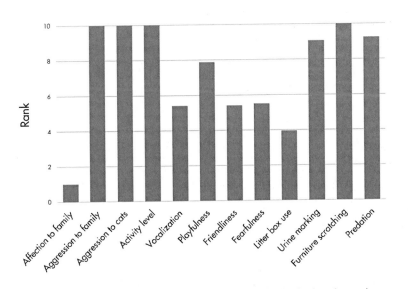

Ranking of the Bengal on the twelve behavioral traits. The higher the ranking, the more likely the cat will exhibit this trait.

Burmese

The Burmese is one of several breeds that takes its name from the country from which it was initially introduced to the United States in 1930. In this case a psychologist, Joseph Thompson, brought the first Burmese, named Wong Mau, into the United States. Wong Mau became the foundation for the Burmese breed in the States. As Thompson suspected, the Burmese was actually a hybrid between the Siamese and an unknown cat of dark color. The name "Burmese" refers to the cat's beautiful and splendid appearance.

While this breed was recognized early on by the CFA, it was one of the breeds that had some difficulty with the registration authorities because it was undergoing continuous crossing between breeds. In 1947 the CFA withdrew its recognition of the Burmese, but recognition was restored in 1953. By now the Burmese has body style characteristics that differentiate it from the Siamese. For one thing, it is considerably heavier than the Siamese, and it has a rounded head that fits with its overall round conformation. American breeders have intentionally bred for a body style that is muscular, almost Bulldog-like, but with a sweet round face with round eyes. In a nutshell the Burmese can be described as a well-rounded cat that is well known for its love of affection. Because of its rather stocky, muscular build, well-rounded eyes, and high ranking in affection, some people refer to their Burmese as their "love bug."

The Burmese comes in a number of color variants, and here is where cat fanciers get a little romantic about their names. You'll find colors such as platinum, lilac, champagne, fawn, chocolate, and cinnamon. Whatever the color, the Burmese short hair coats are relatively low maintenance; stroking the cat often is about all it takes. If you want to go the extra distance you can get a rubber brush to get a little bit better grooming.

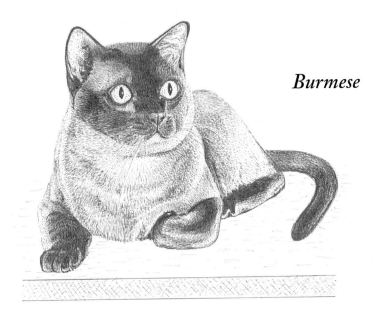

Burmese

Stocky • Muscular • Affectionate • Good litter box use

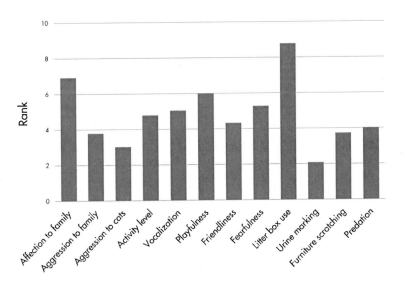

Ranking of the Burmese on the twelve behavioral traits. The higher the ranking, the more likely the cat will exhibit this trait.

You would think that with its Siamese heritage, the Burmese would rank high in vocalization, but it is ranked as average by our authorities. This breed ranks high in affection toward human family members, behind the Ragdoll but higher than the Siamese. To the delight of many Burmese caregivers, its tendency to use the litter box ranks at a high level, and its urine marking tendency is low. This breed is rather moderately ranked in most other traits. A major departure from its Siamese heritage is its lower level of activity. Your Burmese is likely to enjoy curling up in your lap more than climbing on the kitchen shelves.

The Burmese is a breed with a low level of genetic diversity, which results in more frequent occurrences of genetically related diseases. A condition known as the Burmese head defect, which causes episodes of low blood potassium levels (hypokalemia), and gangliosidosis, a neurological disease characterized by muscle tremors and loss of control, are of particular concern. There are genetic tests for these conditions, which should be taken into account during the kitten selection process.

Cornish Rex

If you talk to someone about cats in general, and show them a picture of the Cornish Rex, they're likely to mention something about its alien looks due to its oversized-looking ears, prominent Roman egg-shaped nose, thin boney structure, and unusual wavy hair coat. This breed lacks the outer guard hairs, and even the middle coat of fur seen on most cats, so what is left is a thin undercoat of down. The Cornish Rex looks most like the Sphynx, which even lacks the down layer.

The history of the Cornish Rex is that it was discovered in a litter of kittens born in the 1950s on a farm in Cornwall, England. This breed carries a spontaneous genetic mutation that causes the thin hair coat and whiskers to grow in patterned waves instead of straight, and it is this wavy-hair characteristic that was selected for among early breeders. Geneticists discovered that the gene is recessive; thus, the only way to get the wavy-hair pattern is to breed a male and a female that both have the wavy-hair pattern. The name Rex was borrowed from a breed of rabbits affected by a similar wavy-hair mutation.

The Cornish Rex is renowned for its climbing activity, and some refer to it as the "high flying breed" for its ability to jump from the floor to the caregiver's shoulders in one bounding leap—and enjoy a ride around the house.

It is said that the Cornish Rex is the "greyhound of the cat fancy," referring to its greyhound-like looks and predisposition to be quite active. (But if you want a really active breed, take a look at the Bengal or the Abyssinian.) It ranks on the low side in aggression toward other cats and rather moderately with regard to aggression toward family members, fearfulness of strangers, and vocalization. Urine marking, to the satisfaction of many Cornish caregivers, is at a low level, as is furniture scratching and songbird predation. Litter box use stands out as on the high side.

One thing to keep in mind with the Cornish Rex is the lack of hair coat insulation and the need to keep the environment warm, or at least to provide warm spots. No specific disease vulnerabilities are apparent at this time, but this breed can be particularly susceptible to serious side effects of certain anesthetics; if an anesthetic is needed, advise your veterinarian to err on the side of caution. Because it does not shed fur, the Cornish Rex has a reputation for being hypoallergenic. However, although perhaps not as readily as do most other breeds, it can cause an allergic reaction in some people because the allergens are in the dander, and like all cats the Rex sheds some dander every week. But they are easy to bathe, and therefore the allergens may be held under control.

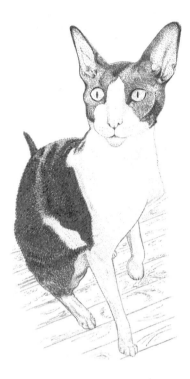

Cornish Rex

- Thin
- Roman nose
- Wavy hair
- Active
- Good litter box use

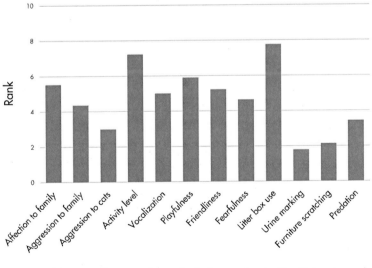

Ranking of the Cornish Rex on the twelve behavioral traits. The higher the ranking, the more likely the cat will exhibit this trait.

Exotic

Despite its name, the Exotic, or what is sometimes called the Exotic Shorthair, is not really all that unusual. In fact, with its appealing teddy bear looks, this is one of the fastest growing breeds in popularity. The Exotic represents an excellent example of an attempt to develop a breed with very specific looks, above all else. Specifically, it is a cat with a Persian head and body shape but with short hair. Persians have about the longest hair of any breed and are known for being rather demanding of upkeep. If you have ever wondered what the Persian looks like underneath all that long hair, take a look at the Exotic. In fact, a good description of the Exotic is that it is a Persian with short hair.

One only gets cats that have a new trait, such as a change in hair coat, by crossing them with another felid, usually other cat breeds or breed types, and in this case it was mostly DSHs that were crossed with Persians. In the CFA a special rule was passed to allow registration to any cat that was a cross between a Persian and a shorthair (while presumably maintaining the Persian body type); thus the door was opened for the Exotic. Because of the much less demanding upkeep in grooming, sometimes the Exotic is referred to as the "lazy man's Persian."

Here is a word about the genetics of shorthair and longhair characteristics. The gene for short hair is dominant over the gene for long hair, which means that since a shorthair cat may carry one short hair and one long hair gene, even two shorthair parents can give rise to longhair offspring. This sometimes surprises the breeder. The Exotic line will remain shorthair as long as one of the parents has two shorthair genes. Although shorthair Exotics can give rise to longhair offspring from time to time, the CFA only accepts the shorthair Exotic for official registration and assigns the longhair to the category of "other."

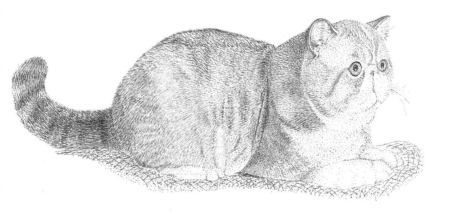

Exotic

Snubby nose • Teddy bear looks • Moderate behavioral traits

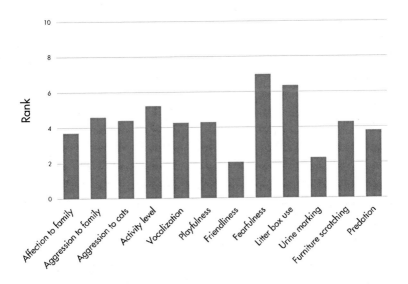

Ranking of the Exotic on the twelve behavioral traits. The higher the ranking, the more likely the cat will exhibit this trait.

The Exotic is known for being heavy boned with the cobby, rounded head of the Persian. This massive head should have a short, snubby, broad nose with a break centered between the eyes. It is said that men who do not like the frou-frou looks of the Persian but who do go for the Persian's rugged, pug-nose face particularly take to them. One authority in the Exotic circle claims that the rapid rise in popularity of this breed is because of the number of two-career couples who, although they like the Persian's looks and personality, are not able to devote the time and upkeep that a Persian requires. Although easily cared for, Exotics are not absolutely carefree and do shed from time to time.

By comparing behavioral profiles, we can see that the activity level of the Exotic is quite a lot higher than that of the Persian. This breed ranks at a rather low level with regard to affection toward family members and is not likely to want to curl up in your lap or be carried around. And like the Persian, the Exotic is moderate in aggression toward human and feline family members, not very friendly to visitors, and ranks high in fearfulness of strangers.

Some have claimed that the reason the Persian does not seem to be as affectionate as other breeds and is not always seeking a warm, cuddly lap, is that with its long hair coat, it easily gets too warm. That this shorthair version of the Persian also ranks below average in affection reveals that this trait is not a function of heating up, but a true behavioral characteristic.

With regard to medical problems, Exotics, like Persians, can be predisposed to polycystic kidney disease. Breeders have worked to identify and eliminate the cats that are positive for this trait. Because of the short nose, and the break between the forehead and just behind the nose, the Exotic, like its Persian cousin, can be susceptible to tearing in the eyes, which requires some attention.

Maine Coon

You may be one of those individuals who live in a family in which one of you wants a cat and the other a dog. If you're looking for a compromise, especially in terms of size, consider the Maine Coon. Females range in size from 9 to 16 pounds, with males running as high as 18 pounds at maturity, larger than many small breeds of dogs. This compromise in choosing the big and brawny cat has settled many a debate. Maine Coons are, in fact, the largest of the purebred cats.

Now, in addition to the large size and heavy build, a characteristic of many individuals in this species is a ringtail, very reminiscent of that of the raccoon. You can imagine how a large cat like this with a raccoon-like tail gave rise to the legend that this breed originated from an accidental cross between a DSH and a raccoon. Not only did the raccoon-like tail contribute to this cat's name, but the paw dexterity of Maine Coons, not unlike that of raccoons, perhaps has added more credibility to the legend. Some Maine Coons even have a fondness for water, which they express by scooping it up with their paws.

For those fanciers of this breed for whom the idea of being hybridized with the raccoon is too far-fetched, the version about Captain Coon of Biddelford Pool, Maine, may be more appealing. The good captain is said to have been very fond of the longhaired cats that he acquired during his travels to and from Europe. The longhaired kittens he brought home were often called "Coon's cats." The mixing of these seafaring cats with the local mousers in Maine are said to have produced the big cats we know today.

The truth of the matter is that longhair cats arrived in the northeastern United States from Europe, and when crossed with local farm cats, some of the larger progeny gave rise to the early Maine Coons. The challenging Maine winters did their own bit of natural selection, and it was the large size and long shaggy coat that repelled water, plus the insulated bushy tail, that helped the fittest Maine Coons survive and outbreed competing cats. In addition, their tufted-hair paws were well suited for negotiating the rugged terrain in snow. The progenitors of this breed were often referred to as Maine Shags because of their full shaggy coats, complete with ear tufts and hair tufts between their toes, and they were renowned for their hunting prowess, and their size. The "coon" part of the name was added on later.

The Maine Coon was registered with the CFA in 1999 and became, for a while, the second most popular cat, after the Persian. This popularity undoubtedly springs from their large size, which has endeared this cat to many. A breed somewhat closely related to the Maine Coon is the Norwegian Forest Cat, which, with its heavy coat and large body size allowing it to withstand harsh winters in Norway, may have even been partially a forerunner to the Maine Coon.

The behavioral profile of the Maine Coon is more or less an exercise in moderation. It ranks second most friendly, right behind the Ragdoll, and very low in fearfulness of strangers, so here is a cat that is likely to approach your visitors, and if they are unsuspecting, do not be surprised if much of the ensuing conversation revolves around the big cat.

The Maine Coon ranks roughly in the upper one third in terms of affection toward family members and fairly low in aggression toward both family members and other cats. It is one of the least vocal breeds.

With regard to maintenance, the first thing to keep in mind is its large size. This means a big scratching post, a big transport carrier, a big litter box, and a big lap for the Maine Coon to sit on. You might think that the long hair coat would create some maintenance problems, but several authorities stated

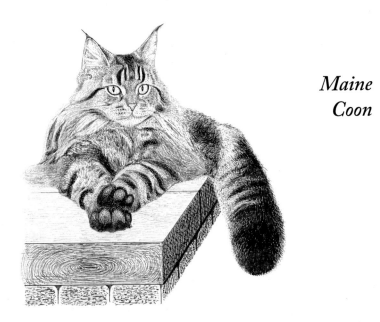

Maine Coon

Largest breed • Affectionate • Friendly • Good litter box use

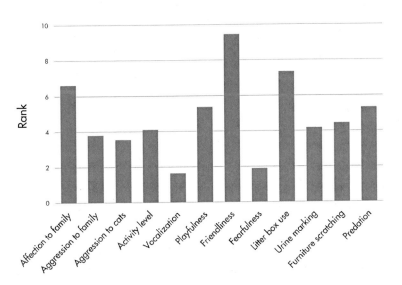

Ranking of the Maine Coon on the twelve behavioral traits. The higher the ranking, the more likely the cat will exhibit this trait.

that this coat is relatively easily maintained. The Maine Coon can be groomed with a medium- to wide-tooth comb and, on occasion, a wire pin brush to prevent matting.

In contrast to the tendency in dogs for the biggest breeds to live the shortest, the Maine Coon lives quite long, fifteen to twenty years. What the large size does create is a susceptibility to hip dysplasia, a joint condition seen in large breeds of dogs, but hardly ever mentioned with regard to cats. The parents of the litter from which you get your Maine Coon should have had their hips screened for hip dysplasia. Maine Coons are also prone to a condition known as hypertrophic cardiomyopathy, so be sure to ask the breeder if the parents of the litter have had their hearts checked for this condition.

Manx

Two things may strike you when you first run across this breed: one is the name, and the other is its uniqueness for being the only breed born without a tail. The name "Manx" refers to the cat's ancestry going back a few hundred years. The Manx was developed as a working farm mouser on the Isle of Man which lies off the coast of England. This is a sturdy breed, strong enough to endure the cold and rainy British weather, and it is known for its hunting skills.

It was in the 1800s that this breed was represented in the first cat show in London, and then they made their way to the United States. The Manx was among the first breeds registered when the CFA was incorporated.

The perfectly rounded rump in your classic Manx is due to the slightly taller hind legs and lack of a tail. With regard to the tailless attribute, there is a variation in the tail within the breed. There are those that have no tail vertebrae at all; those in which you can see, or feel, a small bump where the tail would be; and those in which the tail may be up to an inch long with a few vertebrae. The cats with absolutely no tail are called "rumpy," and the ones with a small bump are called "rumpy-risers." Both of these variants are acceptable for registration and show, but those with a short visible tail, ranging from a bobcat-style to an even longer tail, are not acceptable for show or registration.

Tales about tails: There are interesting stories about how the tailless quality came about. One is that as Noah was closing the door of the ark, and as two lucky cats were allowed in, Noah accidentally closed the door on the cats' tails and ever after this cat was tailless. The other story is that cats were interbred with rabbits and became tailless that way. (The slightly longer hind legs is another trait they share with rabbits.)

Still another fable comes from Celtic folklore. It is said that Celtic warriors added cat tails to their helmets for good luck. In those days tail removal was a bit risky for cats. When a mutation came along for taillessness, these parents were able to reproduce and leave more offspring, so the replacement cats on the Isle of Man became tailless. Regardless of the real tale, it is known that the Manx tailless gene was a spontaneous mutation that occurred on the Isle of Man and then spread throughout the resident cat population.

Examining the behavioral profile, you will see there is still a reflection of the Manx as a working cat; it is not known for being one of the cuddlier breeds, with affection toward family ranking at a low level, and friendliness ranking not much higher. The Manx is a quiet breed, with vocalizations at the lower level. The other behavioral characteristics rank at midrange or just above or below.

The Manx is one of the most long-lived breeds, commonly living twenty years or more. The typical Manx has a short hair coat, but some are longhaired; both types are registered as Manx in the CFA, but in separate divisions.

Because people interested in adopting a Manx expect a completely tailless cat, breeders in the United States may have the tails docked as a kitten. Most breeders will disclose to the pet adopter if the cat has also been surgically docked to assure the typical Manx. The breeding for taillessness seems to be intertwined with some other genetic factors relating to the distal end of the spinal column, and once in a while it can lead to a spinal column defect that can cause incontinence and partial paralysis, which the caregivers will not know about until the cat is around four months of age. You might want to research this further if you are considering choosing a Manx.

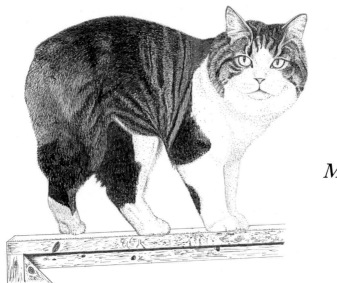

Manx

Tailless • Sturdy • Quiet • Not affectionate

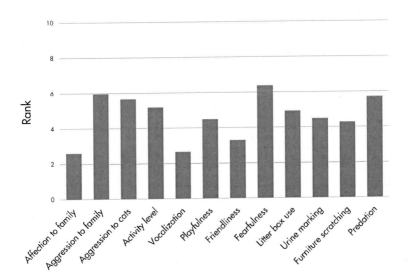

Ranking of the Manx on the twelve behavioral traits. The higher the ranking, the more likely the cat will exhibit this trait.

Norwegian Forest Cat

What you immediately notice in this breed is the dramatic winter coat. Look at a globe and you'll see where this cat originated, and it is not far below the Arctic Circle. The dense, rich fur coat with a wooly undercoat, covered with long guard hairs that are water repellent, has certainly played a role in this cat's popularity and survival in the Nordic area.

In Norse mythology the goddess Freyja, one of the most splendid of the deities, had as her mode of transportation a chariot pulled by two Norwegian Forest Cats. Historians believe that Romans initiated the development of the Norwegian Forest Cat, or "Wegie," by introducing the common European cat to Norway about a thousand years ago, and it wasn't long before the harsh Norwegian climate led to selection of only those cats with long thick coats and rugged bodies that could survive in the northern forest.

Despite its dramatic good looks and the Norse mythology, what you have in the behavioral profile of the Wegie is a cat that ranks as moderate in most traits, with vocalization at the low level.

As for upkeep, Wegies require frequent brushing, especially during the spring when shedding is at its peak. Fortunately the shedding is over with quickly and you do not have to put in this amount of effort throughout the entire year. In the summer the Wegie looks almost like a completely different cat. The shedding of the winter "overcoat" leaves just the short coat with only few vestiges of the winter hair coat grandeur.

With regard to genetically related medical problems, Wegies have a possible glycogen storage disease in certain lines. This rather deadly disease affects the kittens either before they're born or shortly afterward.

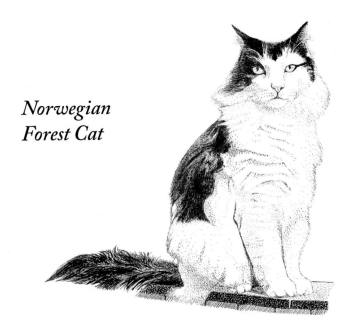

Norwegian Forest Cat

Dramatic winter coat • Moderate in behavioral traits

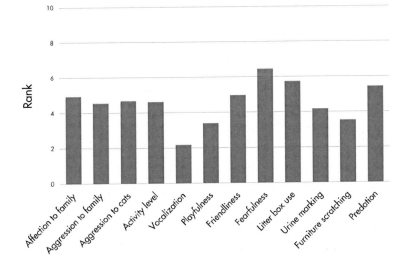

Ranking of the Norwegian Forest Cat on the twelve behavioral traits. The higher the ranking, the more likely the cat will exhibit this trait.

Oriental

The Oriental is a sleek looking, sinuous cat with long tapering lines and a hard muscular body, and some cat fanciers have referred to its svelte body as giving the appearance of agility. Its head is like that of the Siamese, long and wedge-shaped, with straight lines extending into large, flared ears. The Oriental comes in more than 300 colors and typically has short hair with no undercoat. Some variants of this breed have long hair.

In contrast to some other breeds, in which the name reveals the origin, the Oriental did not come from the ancient Orient. Actually, it is not an ancient breed at all, but rather is a newcomer to the cat world, resulting from the handiwork of British breeders who began experimenting with crossbreeding the Siamese back in the 1960s.

Legend has it that Baroness von Ullman of Wolf Springer Cattery in England, while sitting around a warm fire on a cold winter evening in the 1950s, had the vision of developing a breed that looked like a Siamese but did not have the signature coloring or seal point. She tried crossing the seal point Siamese with a Russian Blue, as well as with some other breeds, and eventually created a cat with the body of a Siamese but with a much different hair coat pattern. While intending to retain the Siamese body type and personality, early breeders out-crossed their Orientals with other breeds, including the Abyssinian. As Orientals began trickling into the United States, the breed eventually grew enough in population that in 1977 the Oriental Shorthair was accepted into the CFA. The Oriental Longhair was later accepted.

Read a little bit about the Oriental and you'll find descriptions such as "it moves with athletic grace," "loves attention," "has an irrepressible personality," and "bonds easily with people." Looking at the behavioral profile graph, what you see is

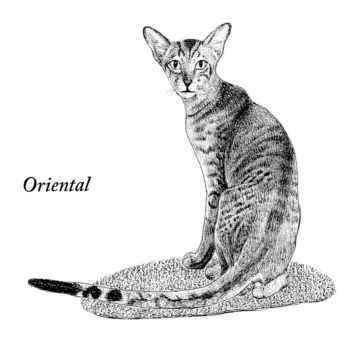

Oriental

Sleek • Sinuous • Muscular • Active • Vocal

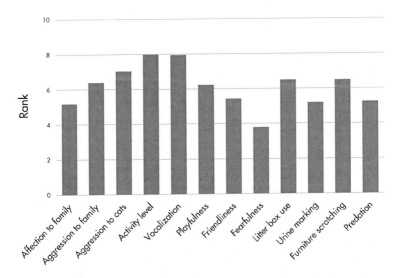

Ranking of the Oriental on the twelve behavioral traits. The higher the ranking, the more likely the cat will exhibit this trait.

a cat that ranks high in activity level and vocalization. As its enthusiasts maintain, the Oriental is a breed with which you need a cat-proof house. And just like its Siamese cousin, it likes to talk. In fact, the only cat that ranks higher on vocalization is the Siamese.

Orientals rank above average in litter box use, and according to our authorities, moderate with regard to urine marking behavior. This breed is moderate in affection toward family members and is less aggressive than the Siamese with both human and feline family members, and according to our authorities it tends to be less fearful. If you're looking for a slim, well-muscled, talkative, affectionate, and active member of the family, the Oriental could be your ideal cat.

As for upkeep, this is one of the more easily cared for cats. Occasional brushing with a rubber brush is usually sufficient to keep it in good shape.

At this time very little seems to be reported with regard to genetically related medical problems, but you should be on the lookout for the same health problems that might plague the Siamese.

Persian

What stands out for this breed is its very distinctive face, and the most distinguishing feature is the deep break just behind the nose that almost makes the profile look like the letter "B." Members of the Persian fan club mention that their large, round eyes give them a very sweet expression, and it's not unusual to hear Persian fanciers refer to them as stunningly beautiful. A bit more straight anatomical talk coming from the CFA refers to the Persian as having a flat face and a stubbed nose. Another distinguishing feature of the Persian is the very long hair. This is a breed that's a medium size with a short, cobby body and heavy boning. The ears are particularly wide set on the head.

The Persian is among the most ancient of cat breeds, and as the name suggests, most authorities believe it originated in and around Persia (now Iran). Others say no one knows for sure, and there are some theories that the breed was developed from generic longhaired cats in Turkey that were crossed with long-hairs in Persia, Burma, China, and Russia. The Persian's initial appearance in Europe was around the sixteenth or seventeenth century. Upon arriving in Europe they enjoyed considerable popularity and, in fact, were part of the first cat show at the Crystal Palace in London in 1871, where they were exhibited under the name "Long-Hair." When it was imported into the United States, and the CFA was launched, the Persian was accepted as one of the initial breeds. Currently the Persian is one of the most popular of the purebred cats in the United States.

Persians come in an array of colors and patterns; among the favored colors are silver and golden. One cat fancier says that when you pair the nice golden color with the aqua colored eyes, the looks are, "just to die for." The lovely eyes have a special feature in that they have a natural mascara, with little black eyelashes and a mascara outline that surrounds the eyes and extends to other parts of the body.

The behavioral profile of the Persian is about as distinctive as its appearance. Perhaps the term used by one Persian enthusiast, "Zen master"—master of the tranquil spirit—says it all. This may be another way of saying that these are quiet cats that enjoy harmony with their families. Take a look at the profile and you will be impressed with all the behavioral traits that would seem to go along with being very laid back and hardly disturbed by anything, as one would expect from a Zen master. While it ranks as moderate in affection, with regard to activity level, vocalization, playfulness, friendliness toward visitors, and even furniture scratching, the Persian ranks the lowest of all the breeds. Persians are known for being rather fearful of visitors (and are ranked very high in this trait by our authorities), which seems to go along with a quiet demeanor. If you want a laid back symbol of peace and tranquility, think of the Persian.

However, keep in mind that your Persian's lack of general activity might extend to the litter box; the Persian ranks the lowest of all breeds in its use. Expect to put an extra bit of effort toward facilitating litter box use, such as finding the favorite type of litter, keeping the box clean, and making it easy to get to, as we discussed in Chapter 4.

Unlike some other breeds, this is not an outgoing cat. However, while only moderately affectionate, your Persian wants to be around you. But take note that there are a couple of precautions to heed. The Persian ranks midway in aggression toward family members and aggression toward other cats. Also, the laid back behavior does not apply to urine marking in that our authorities felt that the Persian could be activated to urine mark in the house, ranking it in the upper one-third of all breeds in this regard. Because interactions with other cats are a primary

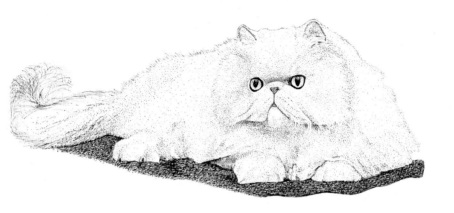

Persian

Distinctive face • Long hair • Inactive • "Zen master"

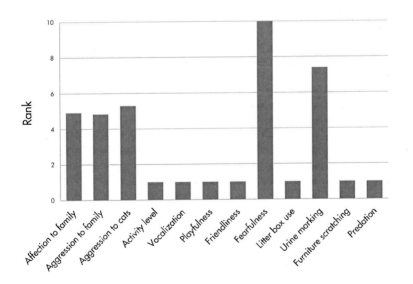

Ranking of the Persian on the twelve behavioral traits. The higher the ranking, the more likely the cat will exhibit this trait.

trigger for urine marking, here is one breed that is a good candidate for being the only cat in the family.

Almost all devoted Persian cat fanciers know that these are high-maintenance animals. It is said that unless you are willing to spend quality time grooming the cat almost every day, this is not the breed for you. Many Persians have constant tears under their eyes, so face washing with a warm washcloth every day to remove this moisture helps quite a bit. Persians have both a cottony undercoat and a silky top coat. The undercoat mats easily and requires upkeep with a metal comb. Most Persian cat caregivers also say that the cat needs a bathing every few weeks. To avoid some of this demanding grooming you could have your Persian's hair clipped to what's called the "lion cut," in which the body is shaved, leaving a fluffy head and tail hair. Here's where it's best to let a professional groomer do the work for you. Recognize, however, that you are not going to convey the sweet, stunningly beautiful Zen master look of this cat if it sports a lion cut. An option to the lion cut is to just clip the cat's underside, which doesn't really change the way it looks, but you're eliminating hairballs in a place where hairball mats are likely to form.

As for genetically related medical problems, cardiomyopathy and polycystic kidney disease are conditions reported for Persians. This is one of the breeds where the polycystic kidney disease is diagnosed in a DNA test, and many breeders have their kittens DNA tested.

Ragdoll

The Ragdoll is one of the newest breeds and one that was developed in the United States, in Southern California. The origin of this breed is attributed to Ann Baker, who happened to notice that one of the offspring of a neighbor's cat seemed to have a very docile predisposition. She bred this cat with one of her Persians and found, to her delight, that the offspring had an exaggerated tendency to go limp in your arms, just like a child's ragdoll. Additional crossbreeding took place with the Burmese and other breeds, with the emphasis always on docility and the love of being handled. The Ragdoll is one of the most recently registered breeds and also one of the fastest growing in popularity, as judged by registration in the CFA. The Ragdoll is even more popular in the United Kingdom and is a rapidly growing breed in the International Cat Association.

The name "Ragdoll" stuck with this breed and perhaps, more than any other breed, the name reflects the behavior. The Ragdoll is probably the best example of intentional development of a cat breed for a particular behavior as a defining endpoint; color and hair coat were of minor concern. Fanciers of this breed like to talk about its tendency to go limp, even to the degree that it can be pushed across the floor as you try to open the door.

You can expect your Ragdoll to greet guests as they come to the door, and even perhaps to be keen on the game of playing fetch. Some authorities say that with the Ragdoll you get puppy-dog-like qualities without having a dog. Others say this breed gives a new meaning to the term "pet under foot." Ragdolls excel at taking it easy. You could even find a number of Ragdolls in a multi-cat household piled on top of each other. A Ragdoll can make an excellent companion for an elderly person who does not want to have an active cat, or for those who do not want a cat that might be knocking valuable knickknacks off the shelf.

One look at the behavioral profile confirms this breed's reputation. Note that the Ragdoll ranks at the bottom in aggression toward family members, aggression toward other cats, and fearfulness exhibited to strangers. And while this breed far exceeds others in affection toward family members (if you leave the room, your Ragdoll could well seek you out and want to be held or petted), you could say that they love socializing with visitors almost as much. They rank tops in friendliness, and may even seem unafraid when being introduced to a dog, so, of course, caution is advised here.

Ragdolls are not very active or vocal and are moderately playful. They rank among the lowest in urine marking, furniture scratching, and songbird predation. Their litter box use is ranked above midway, so you can expect fairly fastidious litter box behavior.

A number of color patterns are found in this breed; perhaps one of the most distinguished is the crème colored cat with Siamese points on the shoulder. Other colors are blue, chocolate, lilac, red, fawn, and cinnamon. The long hair coat is of the non-matting type, but periodic brushing is highly recommended.

This is a breed that takes quite a while to fully mature, and full size isn't reached until the cat is three to four years of age.

In terms of genetically related diseases, this breed is fairly free of most ailments, but a heart disease known as cardiomyopathy is sometimes found. You should find out if the breeder has been testing the parents with ultrasound screening for hypertrophic cardiomyopathy on an ongoing basis.

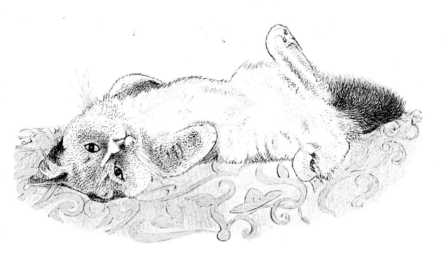

Ragdoll

Relaxed • Affectionate • Friendly • Nonaggressive

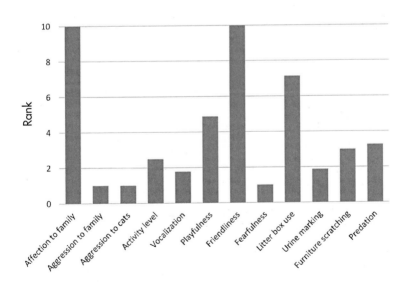

Ranking of the Ragdoll on the twelve behavioral traits. The higher the ranking, the more likely the cat will exhibit this trait.

Russian Blue

Imagine the ballerina of the cat world—lithe, muscular, and elegant—with beautiful green eyes against its grey coat, and you have what fanciers of this breed consider to be unlike any other purebred cat. Now add in a shiny thick hair coat with a luxurious soft feel more or less like silk, and a built-in "smile" that isn't really a smile but rather has something to do with the shape of the face and is nonetheless quite intriguing. It's no wonder that Russian Blue enthusiasts go to some ends to describe this breed's beauty.

The Russian Blue is one of the oldest of the purebreds, with breed recognition in England dating back to the 1800s. The legends surrounding this breed are about as romantic as the descriptions of its beauty. One is that these cats were cherished in the courts of the Russian tsars. Another is that Cossacks carried Russian Blues on their shoulders as they rode into war. The most plausible explanation of the origin of this breed is that in the mid-1800s cats came from Northern Russia on sailing ships bound for England. The thick double coat (this is a cat with which you can trace your initial in its dense coat, and it will remain there until smoothed) was appropriate for this cat, which was adapted to the northern climes.

The name "Russian Blue" has stuck with this breed, which begs the question of why it is called blue when it is really grey. The answer seems to be that grey is not a particularly endearing description for a hair coat color, and breeders preferred the more romantic blue name. Rest assured that your Russian Blue will not have a blue coat and indeed will be a nice shade of grey.

The Russian Blue has been described by enthusiasts as "affectionate, active, playful, at home in an orderly quiet household, and not terribly outgoing." Perhaps this is another way of saying that the behavioral profile of the Russian Blue is re-

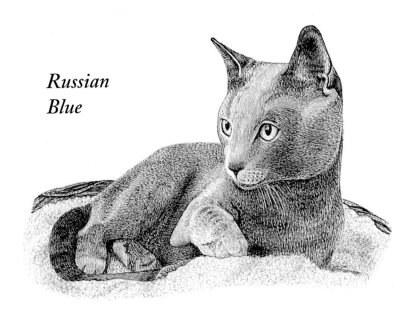

Russian Blue

Lithe • Muscular • Thick coat • Not likely to urine mark • Good litter box use

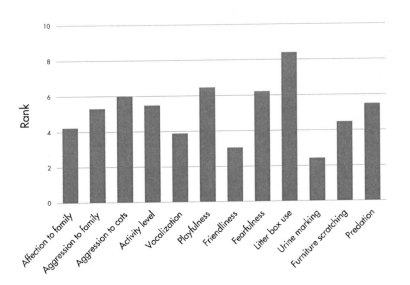

Ranking of the Russian Blue on the twelve behavioral traits. The higher the ranking, the more likely the cat will exhibit this trait.

ally quite moderate in most respects, and a look at the profile graph conveys this description. Two strong positive characteristics are that it ranks high in litter box use and low in urine marking behavior. Russians can be somewhat shy and wary of visitors, but there seems to be a concerted effort to change this through selective breeding.

The thick double coat might lead you to believe that this is a fairly high-maintenance cat, but in fact, fanciers of the Russian Blue feel that it is one of the low-maintenance breeds, where even daily petting seems to do the trick. Just wiping them with a damp cloth will remove the loose hair, and that should be it. To add to the good news, no specific disease vulnerabilities are apparent in this breed at this time.

If a cat with the grace of a ballerina, with one of the sleekest hair coats you could expect to find, plus a very appealing face, and a moderate behavioral profile appeals to you, the Russian Blue could be your ideal cat.

Siamese

Imagine a long, sleek, lithe cat with large pointed ears, almond-shaped blue eyes, and a wedge-shaped head completely relaxed and at home in a palace in ancient Siam. This pretty much epitomizes the vision of this cat, at least to fanciers of the Siamese. This breed originated in Siam (now Thailand), which makes the Siamese one of the most ancient and clearly recognizable breeds in the world, and it has become an icon to cat fanciers and even the public in general. The Siamese was one of the founding breeds of the CFA when it began. With its distinctive markings, color points on the ears, wedge-shaped head, and rather tubular body, the Siamese is immediately recognizable. Some people claim that the Siamese looks very dainty, but then in their next breath tell you that the cat is very muscular.

A Siamese was the personal pet to the royal family of Siam and, as such, enjoyed a life of luxury and pampering. For a period of time the Siamese was, in fact, strictly kept within Siam, and not allowed to leave the country. That's one of the reasons we have little concrete information as to the timeline of development of this breed. As the world got smaller and global trade developed, it became customary for the royalty or dignitaries of one country to present gifts unique to their country to the royalty or dignitaries of the country with which they were doing business. The first Siamese cat that arrived in England in 1884 was a gift from the King of Siam to the English Ambassador to Siam. Not too long after, in the early twentieth century, a Siamese was given to the first lady of the United States, Lady Lucy Webb Hayes, wife of President Rutherford B. Hayes. Not long after the introduction of the Siamese to the world, the breed began to appear in cat shows and grew in popularity to become one of the most favored purebred cats in both the United States and England.

Look at the behavioral profile and you'll see that this breed, while not as docile, affectionate, or nonaggressive as many of its feline counterparts, certainly does not deserve the bad-cat reputation popularized by the Walt Disney movie of the mid-1950s, Lady and the Tramp. This movie featured two Siamese, Si and Am, who slithered and prowled about, vandalizing homes and blaming Lady for all their bad deeds.

Probably the signature behavior of the Siamese is frequent and loud vocalizations; in this it is tops. Siamese aficionados may tell you that the reason they vocalize so much is that they are trying to talk, a reflection of their long history as a companion to human caregivers. Others will tell you that the Siamese helped guard temples and other high places by alerting guards when a stranger was nearing the temple. This may explain why your Siamese likes to climb about and, of course, vocalize—how else would she communicate that there's trouble afoot.

When reading about the Siamese, you get the idea that there is no end to the flattering, descriptive terms used to refer to this breed. Like many breeds, the Siamese is often referred to as having a people personality, craving affection, and thriving on relationships. The well-known vocalization behavior is sometimes referred to as "chitchat," giving a human attribute to this trait.

Siamese do like to move around, ranking behind only the Bengal and Abyssinian in activity level. This breed also ranks high in aggression toward other cats. A problem for some people will be a relatively high ranking in urine marking behavior, and also a high ranking in furniture scratching. What attracts many cat fanciers is that the Siamese has at least a moderate ranking in affection toward family members, playfulness, friendliness toward visitors, and litter box use, and it

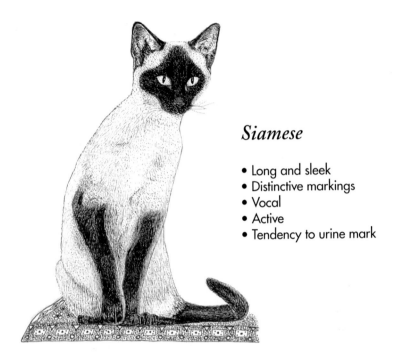

Siamese

- Long and sleek
- Distinctive markings
- Vocal
- Active
- Tendency to urine mark

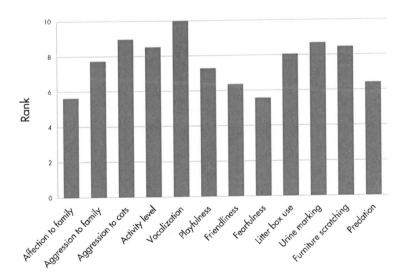

Ranking of the Siamese on the twelve behavioral traits. The higher the ranking, the more likely the cat will exhibit this trait.

is only moderately ranked in predation on songbirds. All in all, this is a behavioral profile that can easily make a cat with a distinctive look and background a very common breed.

With regard to care, Siamese are relatively easy to groom, and with a little brushing, regularly trimming the nails, and cleaning out of the ears, they are what some people call a "wash-and-wear cat." Disease predispositions in this breed are not remarkable.

Sphynx

Here you have a breed that is famous for its attention-getting looks. It is hairless except for a little peach fuzz here and there, and sometimes a few fur tufts, all of which make the ears really stand out. The Sphynx's hairlessness is the result of a gene mutation that was seen in litters from time to time around the world. Thus, tracking down the particular progenitors of the Sphynx before the mutation occurred is difficult. One version of the origin of the Sphynx is that the breed developed when two hairless female kittens were born, and the breeder, in turn, bred these with a Devon Rex, and perhaps some other shorthair breeds. The hairless trait continued in those selected as the founders of the breed.

The name "Sphynx" has nothing to do with the breed being of Egyptian origin, but can be traced back to a CFA member, David Mare, who in 1973 said when he first saw this cat that he was reminded of an Egyptian cat statue in the Louvre, which he thought bore a resemblance to the breed. Mr. Mare of course knew that the actual sphinxes in the valley of the Nile were not cats, but he thought nonetheless that "Sphynx" would make a wonderful breed name, and the name stuck.

There are several things to say about the hairless characteristic. When you pet the Sphynx, the skin feels quite different than that of other cats. Because it lacks a hair coat, this cat requires a warm environment, and you are likely to find that your Sphynx wants to cuddle up quite often to keep warm. Your initial impression might be that this is a low maintenance pet. However, the oil produced in its skin is not absorbed by fur and therefore tends to be deposited on furniture, as well as on laps. Also, the oily skin acts like a magnet for grime and dirt and may leave a dirty spot where the Sphynx regularly lies on bedding or furniture. So, instead of the fur grooming that is required for many breeds, the maintenance is soapy washing, every week or so.

Another misconception about the Sphynx is that these cats are hypoallergenic. Because they still produce dander proteins and therefore have dander in their saliva from grooming, like other cats they are allergenic to those susceptible because it is the dander proteins that are allergy producing. However, there is an upside to having a hairless cat: There are no hairballs to worry about, no shedding, and happily, no fleas.

Looking at this cat, you might feel that it is perhaps skittish, a bit wild, and unfriendly, but in fact, fans of this breed refer to the Sphynx as loving and patient, which is reflected in the behavioral profile as moderately affectionate and relatively low in aggression toward family members. They are also moderately playful. They rank low in friendliness toward visitors, although they are not particularly fearful.

Give the Sphynx high scores in the household sanitation area; they are ranked as the least likely of all breeds to engage in urine marking behavior and are near the top in litter box use. And their low ranking in furniture scratching is another house-friendly trait.

Because the Sphynx has ties to the minimal-haired Devon Rex and Cornish Rex breeds, you should be aware of the possibility of serious side effects to certain anesthetics known for affecting the Rex cats, and if an anesthetic is needed, advise the veterinarian to be cautious. Other than this concern, and perhaps a bit counterintuitive given the looks of the Sphynx, no particular disease predispositions are apparent at this time.

What it all boils down to with the Sphynx is appreciating their unique looks and family-friendly behavioral profile. We encourage you to get an Egyptian cat statue to be reminded of the rather roundabout way your Sphynx got its name.

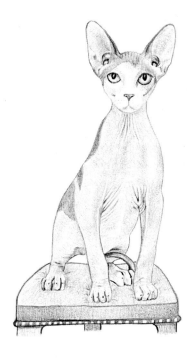

Sphynx

- Hairless
- Oily skin
- Playful
- Least likely to urine mark
- Good litter box use

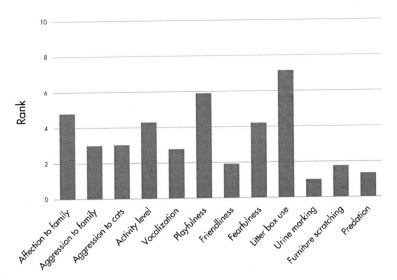

Ranking of the Sphynx on the twelve behavioral traits. The higher the ranking, the more likely the cat will exhibit this trait.

Tonkinese

In numerous articles in Cat Fancy and other publications, writers exuberantly talk about how the Tonkinese makes an ideal pet, stating that this breed gets along with children and is friendly to other cats. One fancier characterizes it as "a rather chatty breed," which makes sense because the Tonkinese is ranked just behind Siamese and Oriental in vocalization. Another fancier gives the vocalization tendency a romanticized twist, describing these cats as "smooth talkers."

The Tonkinese was the result of rather enterprising breeders in Canada in the 1960s who started breeding Siamese with Burmese and ended up with a cat that is intermediate in body size and more stocky than the Siamese. While one of the breeders initially suggested the name "Tonkanese," the name Tonkinese was settled upon, reflecting this cat's ancestral origins in Burma (Burmese) and Siam/Thailand (Siamese) and their proximity to the Gulf of Tonkin. This choice of name was probably influenced by the prevalence of the Gulf of Tonkin name during the Vietnam War in the 1960s. The name stuck, and the Tonkinese was registered with the Canadian Cat Association (CCA) in 1971 and the CFA in 1978. Tonkinese come in four base coat colors (platinum, champagne, natural, and blue) and three coat patterns (point [like the Siamese], mink, and solid [like the Burmese]).

Over the years the Tonkinese has grown in popularity. This breed ranks fairly high in affection, activity level, vocalization, playfulness, and friendliness and low in fearfulness. And, according to our authorities, the Tonkinese excels at litter box use and has a low tendency to urine mark, more similar to the Burmese than the Siamese, which ranks high in urine marking behavior. If you want an active, playful,

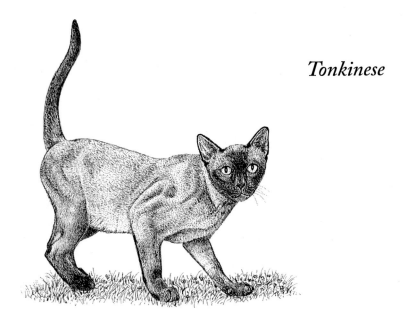

Tonkinese

Well built • Friendly • Not likely to urine mark • Good litter box use

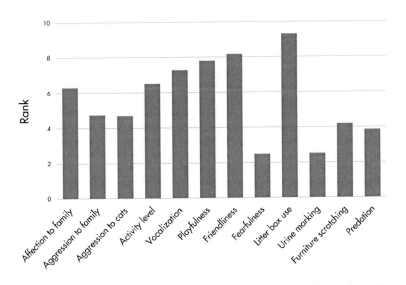

Ranking of the Tonkinese on the twelve behavioral traits. The higher the ranking, the more likely the cat will exhibit this trait.

affectionate cat that feels free to vocalize and is friendly to visitors, the Tonkinese is a breed certainly worth considering as your ideal cat.

Regarding upkeep and maintenance, caregivers of the Tonkinese are the first to say that this is one of those "wash-and-wear" breeds that is relatively low maintenance, maybe requiring once-a-week brushing. Perhaps because this is a new breed, without a long history in breed restriction, there seem to be no particular disease predispositions that are apparent, other than a gum condition, gingivitis, which seems to plague the Oriental breeds and merits attention. Who knows, you may want to take up the challenge of trying to brush your cat's teeth. Good luck.

Domestic shorthair

We cannot talk about cat breeds without discussing the generic and most common domestic cat, the one that is virtually treated as a breed—the domestic shorthair (DSH). The longhaired cousin of the DSH is referred to as the domestic longhair (DLH). (Domestic medium hair [DMH], the name for the medium length hair coat style, is a term much less used.) The DSH is almost always the cat you see featured in magazine or television ads when cats are used to help promote products. (This is not so with dogs: almost all dogs used in advertising are of an identifiable breed.)

We cannot refer to the DSH without mentioning the closely related American Shorthair, which is a purebred cat and one of the original breeds accepted by the CFA back in 1906. The American Shorthair, which we do not cover as a separate breed in this book, actually arose from early DSH farm and house cats when a group of breeders wanted to consolidate what they thought were the most desirable morphological characteristics and started selecting for a cat that bred true to their expectations. The American Shorthair is said to be one of the two breeds native to the United States, sharing this distinction with the Maine Coon. The American Shorthair comes in a variety of colors, and the DSH an even greater variety.

To explain a little bit more, cats originally arrived in the United States from Europe by boat (including on the Mayflower). These cats were used to keep down rodents on the ships, and then around the farms in the New World. Apparently an offshoot of the British Shorthair, these cats were fairly uniform in body style. Eventually these cats were bred with Siamese and Persians, which introduced quite a bit of variability. Mostly the scales tipped in favor of those who really liked the looks of the British Shorthair.

In the DSH you will see a good deal of variety, reflecting crossbreeding that produces litters that can be quite diverse. In this book we provide a behavioral profile of the DSH that our authorities felt was fairly representative of the typical short-hair found in most homes and animal shelters. DSHs have also found their way into our lives as feral cats fed by cat lovers throughout the world.

Turn to the DSH behavioral profile graph and you find a relatively moderate profile with strong rankings in affection toward family, playfulness, friendliness, and activity level. Aggression toward family members is in the upper one-half of breeds, as is aggression toward other cats. There are two elements to focus on in the behavioral profile. One is that the DSH seems to have retained its strong instinct for sanitary behavior, being ranked tops with regard to litter box use. But note also that this is the top-ranked breed for urine marking behavior. This can be a serious concern, especially if you are planning to get a male cat, because males, neutered or not, are much more likely to urine mark in the house than females, and this includes even males neutered as early as eight weeks of age. If you really want to reduce the chance of urine marking by a cat in your home, consider a female. You can also look at breeds that rank much lower on urine marking.

Finally, the DSH is your classic songbird predator. If you are concerned about doing everything you can to keep songbirds around your property, especially those young fledglings, consider making your DSH an indoor-only cat. If you enjoy a garden with songbirds and still want your cat to be outdoors some, there are other breeds that rank much lower in this trait.

The genetically related disease predispositions listed in the purebred profiles are specific to each particular breed. Because the DSH is, by definition, not a purebred, we cannot point to particular disease vulnerabilities. This should not be taken to imply that the DSH does not have genetically related disease vulnerabilities, but that these are on a case-by-case basis.

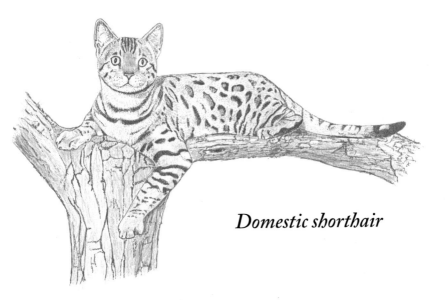

Domestic shorthair

- Not a purebred—physical and behavioral traits vary
- Tendency to urine mark but good litter box use

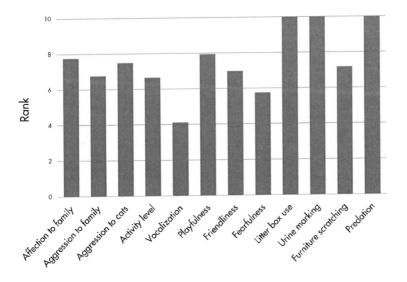

Ranking of the domestic shorthair on the twelve behavioral traits. The higher the ranking, the more likely the cat will exhibit this trait.

Domestic longhair

This cat is the longhaired cousin of the DSH. African wild cats, the main progenitors of the modern domestic cat, were all shorthairs. However, hair coat mutations occur from time to time. The gene responsible for long hair is recessive, meaning that any particular cat needs two copies of this gene in order to have long hair. Hence, longhaired cats are much less common than shorthaired cats.

There has been a good deal of interest on the part of cat historians as to the origin of the longhair characteristic and how it became widespread. Some trace it back to Persian ancestry and the introduction of longhaired Persian cats to Europe that in turn bred with the resident shorthairs. Others say that the longhair mutation arose at the same time in three different areas: Russia, Persia, and Turkey. Still others say that the longhair mutation originated in Russia, where in the Siberian winter, the hair coat would serve any cat well in terms of survival. From Russia this longhair cat then spread into Turkey and Persia, giving rise to the longhair cats from these regions.

Regardless of the true story, longhair cats were first seen in Europe in the 1500s, originally in Italy and then in France. Sometimes they were given the nickname "angora," referring to the old Turkish city of Angora (now Ankara). From France they then reached Britain. Somewhere around the mid-nineteenth century, cat enthusiasts began distinguishing the Turkish angora cats from other longhair cats coming from Persia and Russia.

In this book we deal with a number of breeds that have both shorthair and longhair versions. The DLH historically represents a mixture of breedings of several types of longhair cats, where from time to time the recessive gene crops up. This happens often enough that even DSH breedings can result in longhair (DLH) cats.

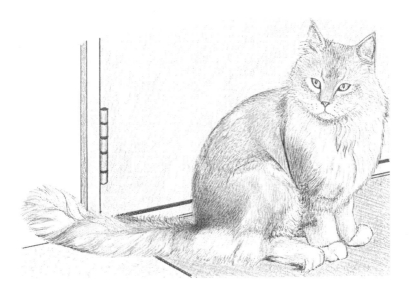

Domestic longhair

- Not a purebred—physical and behavioral traits vary
- Tendency to urine mark but good litter box use

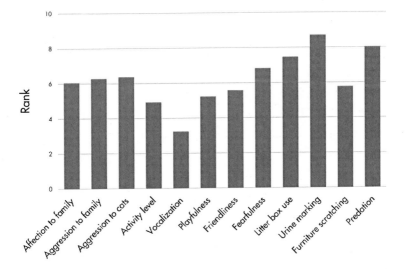

Ranking of the domestic longhair on the twelve behavioral traits. The higher the ranking, the more likely the cat will exhibit this trait.

Interestingly, there is no corresponding CFA-recognized breed to the DLH like the American Shorthair counterpart to the DSH. In the cold climates such as Maine, Alaska, and northern Minnesota, longhair cats have a definite survival advantage, and this has been the secret to the well-established permanency of long hair in some of the breeds.

Turning to the behavioral profile, what we see is a slightly moderated version of the shorthair profile, with urine marking third from the highest, behind the DSH and the Bengal. The ranking in litter box use is somewhat below that of the DSH. The DLH is also ranked somewhat lower than the shorthair version with regard to affection and aggression, activity level, vocalization, furniture scratching, and even predation.

Keep in mind that the very longhaired cats do not make good outside animals because their hair coats are very prone to matting, and being outdoors tends to make upkeep more difficult. There are authorities that say they should be groomed for half an hour per day, which probably exceeds the time budget of many would-be caregivers. At any rate, there is a definite tradeoff. In looking at the DLH as your new feline housemate, keep hair coat maintenance in mind. As mentioned for the DSH, this breed is, by definition, not a purebred, and we cannot point to particular disease vulnerabilities. Some individual DLH cats may well have genetically related disease vulnerabilities, but these are on a case-by-case basis.

Chapter 8

Why cats do that: Purring, yawning, eating grass, and flipping out on catnip

This chapter applies to all breeds and both genders. It is about the intriguing things that cats do that endear them to us, make us wonder about cat behavior, and even entertain us. We are enthusiastic about ending this book by addressing the question we often ask about our cats: Why do they do that? We have one caveat, however, regarding the explanations we provide as to why cats purr, yawn, munch on grass, and flip out on catnip. The research is not yet definitive and is still ongoing; our interpretations fit best with the science available and seem to make the most sense. Ten years from now we could be adjusting, or at least fine-tuning, some explanations.

Why cats purr

Perhaps the most unique and endearing behavior of cats is purring. But why do cats purr? Dogs don't, horses don't, sheep don't, people don't. But some animals, such as other felids, do purr—we'll get to that. The next question is, how do cats purr?

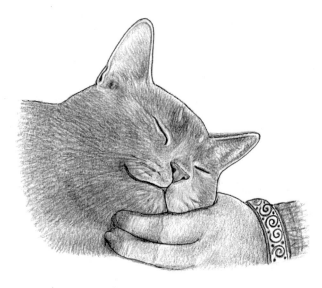

Yes, a purring kitty can make it look like purring is all about contentment, but there is more to it than that. The low-pitched 25 Hz fundamental frequency of purring appears to play a role in wound healing and maintaining muscular and bone strength.

As it turns out, new answers to these questions have recently emerged due to the curiosity of scientists. First, here is a bit on the mechanism of how cats purr. Recordings show that purring is produced by a signal originating in the brain, innervating muscles of the larynx, causing muscle twitches at the rate of 25 cycles per second (25 hertz [Hz]), which produce a vibration at the same frequency. Because this is such a low frequency vibration, what we hear is a harmonic, that is, a multiple of the basic 25 Hz, such as 50 Hz or 100 Hz. However, the cat actually feels the 25 Hz vibrations. Interestingly, purring occurs during both inspiration and expiration. And, cats can purr while they meow. Kittens purr at the same low frequency as adult cats; size makes no difference.

While you might think of purring as a way of communicating a feeling of contentment, that is not the complete picture.

An insight into the reason cats purr comes from research on the use of low frequency vibrations, around the 25 Hz frequency just mentioned, by physical therapists on humans for promoting wound healing, relieving pain, increasing muscle mass, and helping in the repair of tendons and muscles. It is postulated that the same effects on muscles and bones can occur in cats during purring. When a wild felid goes for the all-out chase for a dinner, and comes back with sore muscles and overly stretched tendons, purring is healing.

Veterinarians are well aware that cats frequently purr when injured or sick—even on the exam table. And they often purr when giving birth. While these examples certainly do not represent contentment, neither do they mean that the sick or injured cat that purrs is psychotic. According to the hypothesis here, cats are using the instinctual behavior inherited from their wild ancestor that promotes body healing. The sick or injured cat that purrs is a smart cat. And yes, there is an advantage to mothers purring with their kittens; it likely helps the mother to recover from the trauma of giving birth and the kittens to grow stronger bones.

Aside from helping to repair injured tissue, purring also has a function of preserving muscle mass and bone strength. Cats purr a lot while just lying around—undoubtedly even when we do not know about it. While felids are your prototypical couch potato, they do not lose muscle mass and body condition from doing nothing like us humans. Would that we mere humans could purr!

What felids purr? Since the writings of Darwin it has been known that several wild felids, including pumas, cheetahs, and ocelots, purr. Darwin believed that lions, jaguars, and leopards do not purr. Here again, Darwin was right. Research has added bobcats, lynx, and the African wild cat ancestor of the domestic cat to the list of purrers, and tigers to the list of nonpurrers. The large felids that purr do so at about the same 25 Hz frequency as the domestic cat.

As to why some felids purr and others do not, we can point to the interesting fact that those felids that purr cannot roar, and those felids that roar cannot purr. It boils down to the degree of ossification in the bones of the larynx (the hyoid apparatus, to be exact). To make a long anatomy lesson short, the species with a fully ossified, or stiff, hyoid apparatus purr and they thus enjoy the purring-related health benefits. The species with a non-ossified, elastic, hyoid apparatus roar but can't purr or enjoy the benefits of purring. Look at it this way, if roaring good and loud gets you your way more often with regard to resources in nature, you must give up the benefits of purring. Like most things in life, felids can't have it both ways.

Why cats yawn

Here is a behavior that we share not only with our cats, but our dogs, horses, cows, sheep, and even birds. We can look at why we yawn to come up with insights.

According to the leading old-school theory, we yawn because of a low oxygen level in the blood, and yawning opens up the aerating sacs (alveoli) of the lungs and oxygenates the blood. The theory goes that when our animals (or we) are inactive, such as just before going to sleep, or upon waking up, our lungs have not been fully used and the "involuntary" yawn fills unused alveoli, getting them active again and increasing blood oxygen levels up to normal. The problem is, blood oxygen and carbon dioxide levels are the same in sleepy as fully awake animals, and if you administer oxygen to the sleepy person or animal, yawning still occurs. Besides, unborn fetuses even yawn. Yawning, as it turns out, has nothing to do with oxygenating the blood.

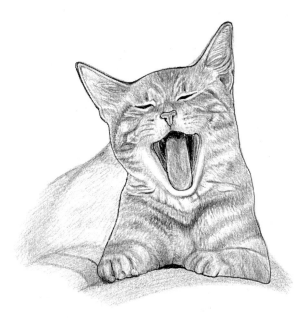

Look familiar? Cats yawn just like us—upon awakening and when drowsy. Yawning has nothing to do with oxygenating the blood. It is now believed that yawning activates a sleepy brain, presumably by cooling it via the vascular supply.

Recently, researchers put forth the theory that what yawning really does is activate the brain, and it does this primarily by cooling the brain. When we, or our cats, are inactive, such as when just waking up or while resting—or in the human instance, listening to a boring talk—the blood flow to the brain slows down. Since the brain produces more heat than the rest of the body, a good blood flow is essential because the blood pulls heat from the brain, keeping it from overheating. When we are resting or being bored and the blood flow slows a bit, the brain tends to heat up.

Now the brain, like any high-powered computer, works best when cooler. When we, or our cats, are sleepy, a good yawn increases the blood-cooling mechanism, revving up the computer, and we can put off sleeping a while. The same thing happens upon awakening, when the brain needs a boost. The cooling of the brain by blood flow requires that the blood is cooled before it enters the brain, and this happens primarily by cooled venous blood coming from the nasal area, cooling arterial blood coming in around the base of the brain. Yawning, with the jaws held open for a few seconds, helps to cool this nasal venous blood.

In humans, great apes, and possibly dogs, yawning is catching—you yawn, I yawn. While no one has shown that dogs "catch" the yawns of other dogs, there is some good evidence that dogs can catch human yawns. We do not know about cats catching yawns of other cats or their human caregivers. With humans there is also the notion that yawning reflects some empathy with fellow humans, while others claim that by catching another's yawn, you are getting your brain activated too, just in case something dangerous is around the corner.

Why cats eat grass and houseplants

If you have been around cats much when they have access to grass or houseplants, you probably have seen them munching away. Both cats and dogs are commonly observed to eat grass and other plant items that have no nutritional value. The explanations have often been that plants provide fiber or that the animal is feeling ill and eating grass induces them to vomit. If you have seen cats eat grass, it is likely that you have not detected any signs of illness and have not seen them vomit regularly afterward.

So what is the explanation for grass and plant eating? For one thing, it is known that wild felids and canids in nature are known to eat grass. For example, grass is seen in 5 to 10 percent of the scats of cougars and wolves. Most domestic cats eat grass as their preferred plant.

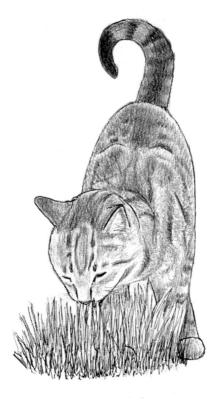

Plant eating, especially grass eating, is a behavior seen in other felid species. Plant eating a few times a week is a normal behavior of healthy cats and seems to be related to an instinct inherited from ancestral cats living in the wild that serves to keep intestinal worms to a minimum.

To get more information on plant eating by cats from hundreds of caregivers in a position to observe who, where, and when their cats ate plants, we launched a web-based survey and got close to 1,500 useable survey responses on both outdoor and strictly indoor cats. We particularly focused on whether caregivers observed signs of sickness before their cats ate grass, signs of vomiting afterward, and diet.

Grass was the most frequently eaten plant, but not the only plant eaten. Contrary to popular belief, only about 10 percent of cat caregivers reported that their cats frequently show signs of illness prior to plant eating, and only 20 percent reported that their cats regularly vomit afterward. Therefore, we conclude that grass and plant eating is not related to illness, and only sometimes is followed by vomiting. And we found no relationship between type of diet and plant eating, which does not lend support to the dietary fiber idea.

The best explanation for grass and plant eating is that this is a normal behavior, not associated with illness or a dietary need but an instinctual predisposition, inherited from wild felid ancestors. In nature, felids are always exposed to intestinal parasites, so basically all wild cats carry some intestinal parasite load. There is reason to believe, especially based on research on wild chimpanzees, that grass eating has an intestinal parasite purging effect. That is presumably why cougars regularly eat grass. Grass eating is a type of self-medication—herbal medicine if you will. Grass and plants are nature's deworming medicine.

One more interesting finding is that young cats, those less than one year of age, eat grass more frequently than do adult cats. The explanation for this is that in nature, young, rapidly growing felids are more vulnerable than adult cats to intestinal parasites that steal nutrition. So, having an instinctive drive to eat grass for intestinal parasite purging makes sense.

Here are some practical precautions to take. For one thing, chemicals applied to lawns can be toxic. You might control what is put on your lawn and restrict the cat's access for a bit after spraying; of course you do not necessarily know about the neighbor's lawn. This is another reason to have the cat live indoors only. However, the indoor environment has its risks too. Many houseplants are toxic to cats. If your cat has the perfectly normal drive to eat plants, and grass is not available, the cat may turn to munching one of your houseplants. Not that the houseplants are likely to be fatal if eaten, but they can cause vomiting, diarrhea, excessive salivation, and irritation of the lips. So here is a good reason to provide your indoor cat with a grass garden: you humor their instinct and provide an appealing alternative to houseplants, toxic or not.

Even with an indoor grass garden, some cats may experiment a bit and try a houseplant also. This is especially true of young cats, or even kittens, that are drawn to more of a variety of plants to eat. Be vigilant and keep the houseplants out of reach. Here is a list of some of the poisonous plants:

Azalea/Rhododendron	Marijuana
Amaryllis	Peace Lily (Mauna Loa
Autumn Crocus	Peace Lily)
Castor Bean	Oleander
Chrysanthemum	Pothos
Cyclamen	Sago Palm
English Ivy	Schefflera
Kalanchoe	Tulip/Narcissus Bulbs
Lilies	Yew

If you suspect that your cat (or dog) has eaten a poisonous plant, call your veterinarian and the ASPCA Animal Poison Control Center hotline (888-426-4435).

Why cats flip out on catnip

All cat caregivers know that many cats love catnip, or seem to, and even flip out over it. Why is this? Do all felids respond this way? Is there some adaptive function? Are they reacting to what they smell, or is it a marijuana-like reaction to the catnip they consume? As it turns out, here is a behavior in which we cannot point to a possible adaptive benefit; the behavior seems to have no evolutionary survival value. However, the behavior is "normal" in the sense that lots of cats react to catnip, and it is not related to any medical problem.

Here are some useful insights into this strange, felid-specific behavior. First of all, only 50 to 70 percent of cats respond to catnip. For those that do, the catnip reaction typically involves sniffing and then chewing the catnip source, generally a cloth mouse stuffed with dry catnip leaves. However, cats respond to catnip no matter how it is packaged, or whether the leaves are freshly picked or dried. The initial reaction to the catnip may progress to rubbing their chins or cheeks on the source, and rubbing their bodies on the ground alongside the mouse, reminiscent of female courtship behavior. Some cats progress to batting the mouse like a kitten playing with a leaf. Also common is pawing and digging at the mouse with the hind legs, and/or biting into it—behaviors that are very like the way a cat bites into a rodent prey. These catnip reactions occur more or less at random. Then there is a satiation effect, so that the reaction lasts only five to fifteen minutes and cannot be evoked again for an hour or so.

Scientists have discovered that the active ingredient that cats respond to is a type of lactone called nepetalactone. At this point, the best explanation for the array of responses is that catnip activates different areas of the brain that control female courtship-like behavior, kitten-like play, and predatory behavior, at random. We know from research that the catnip reaction is mediated by the sense of smell; catnip does not have to be ingested, and is usually not eaten.

Are domestic cats the only species that respond to catnip? As it turns out, several felids other than domestic cats are known to flip out on catnip: lions, leopards, jaguars, bobcats, pumas, and ocelots.

So how did cats and catnip get together? You would think that if cats and other responding felids grew up and lived where

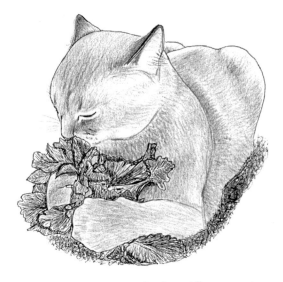

Cats and their beloved at catnip evolved on different continents; they met up in Europe and North America by accident. The attraction of cats to all forms of catnip seems to be incidental. There is no adaptive function to cats' flipping out on catnip, for cats or the plant.

catnip grows they would be always tripping out—kittens would be neglected, cats would lose their edge in hunting, and the catnip lovers might lose their territory. Not surprisingly then, the catnip plant (*Nepeta cataria*) and the ancestral domestic cat and other felid species that respond to this plant are native to different continents. Catnip is native to Eurasia, and the catnip-responding felids are native to North, Central, and South America and sub-Saharan Africa. Interestingly, the tiger, which is native to Eurasia, where catnip originated, does not respond to catnip.

Enter the human factor. People have transported both cats and the catnip plant around the world: We humans brought cats and catnip together. The catnip reaction appears to be an incidental, functionless result of our mingling with nature. Now cats have access to the plant if it is provided by human caregivers.

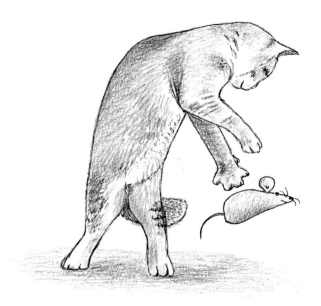

The strange reaction of cats to a catnip mouse or loose catnip leaves seems to result from the random activation of neural circuits associated with courting, play, and predation behaviors.

Here is a new twist to the catnip story, presented here as a mere possibility. Based on how a cat often bats around and "plays" with a real mouse it has just caught, in a catnip-like fashion, it is quite plausible that there is a connection between the effects of catnip and the effects of mice on cats. Mice are known to produce lactones in skin secretions, especially when they are stressed. It is likely that the lactone secretion of a stressed mouse is enough like nepetalactone, that when mice are caught and stressed by a cat, they produce this secretion and the cat goes through a "catnip reaction" that distracts them from the mouse long enough to give the mouse a chance to escape. This catnip-mimic secretion would be the mouse's "magic potion," offering a last chance to escape. No wonder dried catnip is almost always packaged as a cloth mouse.

Epilogue

The popularity of cats in American homes, and in those in other developed countries around the world, has grown to the point that cats now outnumber dogs as the most common human companion animal. The reasons are numerous, but certainly a big factor is that in the modern era we are away from our homes many more hours during the week and our living spaces are smaller. This makes cats the perfect companion animal. But we, as caregivers, differ in what we value in a cat.

The close proximity with which cats share our lives, and the rather long duration of their time with us—sometimes as much as twenty years—means that their behavior impacts us and affects what we gain personally from this relationship. In this book we discussed how recognized breeds, as well as the sexes, can differ substantially in their everyday behavior. By presenting this data our intention was not to gloss over the importance of individual differences within a breed or gender.

Rather, the profiles in this book are generalizations that point to major differences between the breeds and genders.

Given what cats can mean to us, and how we differ in what we find most rewarding in our experiences with them, our goal with this book was to provide you with breed and gender behavioral profiles that will help you to select the cat best suited to your personality, lifestyle, and home environment. Welcoming a new kitten or cat into your home is an important step. We trust that our tips may make that transition easier for you and your new companion, and that our thoughts on raising cats to encourage the behaviors we like and discourage those we do not like may also prove to be useful. We hope we have helped you find and enjoy the friendship of *your ideal cat.*

Annotated bibliography

I. General books about cats

Clutton-Brock, J. *Cat.* New York: Dorling Kindersley, 1991.

> Clutton-Brock contributes to the DK Eyewitness Books, almost equally focusing on wild and domestic cats. Each topic gets two pages, for example, cat characteristics; shorthairs; longhairs; caring for your cat, which depicts the items required for cat care.

Edwards, A. *The Ultimate Encyclopedia of Cats, Cat Breeds & Cat Care.* London: Hermes House, 2006.

> This book comprehensively discusses care of cats and then introduces the longhair, semi-longhair, and shorthair groups of breeds, as well as the non-pedigreed cats. The beautiful photographs clarify specific behaviors and techniques of care.

Hart, B. L., L. A. Hart, and M. J. Bain. *Canine and Feline Behavior Therapy.* 2nd ed. Ames, IA: Blackwell, 2006.

This is a comprehensive text meant for veterinarians that deals with problem behaviors of cats as well as dogs, by providing background information and then discussing the diagnosis of problem behaviors, followed by treatment guidelines. Two chapters are devoted to the interactions of pets with their human companions, emphasizing the benefits of pets to human mental and physical health, and dealing with pet loss.

Hofmann, H. *The Natural Cat: Understanding Your Cat's Needs and Instincts: Everything You Should Know about Your Cat's Behavior.* Stillwater, MN: Voyageur Press, 1994.

Hofmann begins with cats depicted in religion and art, as well as their evolution. Most of the book is devoted to the behaviors of cats from an everyday perspective: eating and drinking, grooming, sleeping, courtship, and old age.

Leyhausen, P. *Cat Behaviour: The Predatory and Social Behavior of Domestic and Wild Cats.* New York: Garland STOM Press, 1979.

Leyhausen's classic work is famous for its diagrammatic illustrations of offensive and defensive body postures and facial expressions of cats. Anyone interested in predatory or social behavior of cats will enjoy reading this book.

II. Choosing and welcoming your kitten

Hart, B. L., and R. A. Eckstein. "The Role of Gonadal Hormones in the Occurrence of Objectionable Behaviours in Dogs and Cats." *Applied Animal Behaviour Science* 52 (1997): 331–344.

This research paper notes that experience and age at the time of castration do not predict which cats or dogs will be affected by castration.

Siino, B. S. *The Complete Idiot's Guide to Choosing a Pet*. New York: Alpha Books, 1999.

This book considers a variety of pets and presents a shopping list of essential supplies for each. The author scores cats as midrange on the time commitment required, with fairly easy feeding and cleanup. They are scored moderate on suitability with children five years and older, and low for children under five years of age. Based on the information in this book, some breeds that are high on affection and low on aggression may work out quite well with young children.

III. Historical background of the domestic cat

Even though the cat is the world's most popular pet, only recently have scientists begun putting together the ancient origin and developmental history of the domestic cat. Judging by the cat images in ancient Egyptian artwork, we all assumed that Egyptians were the first to keep cats as pets, starting around 3,600 years ago. Recent advances in deciphering the feline genome reveal that domestication actually began about 10,000 years ago in the Middle East. A rather touching picture of the ancient domestication that fits the DNA data was the discovery of a 9,500-year-old burial site on the island of Cyprus, where an adult person was laid to rest in a grave together with an 8-month-old cat. The human and cat were oriented in the same direction, revealing a bond between them. Read more about the origin of the domestic cat in the following sources.

Clutton-Brock, J. *Cats: Ancient and Modern*. Cambridge: Harvard University Press, 1993.

Driscoll, C. A., J. Clutton-Brock, A. C. Kitchener, and S. J. O'Brien. "The Taming of the Cat." *Scientific American* 300, no. 6 (2009): 68–75.

Kitchener, A. *The Natural History of the Wild Cats.* Ithaca, NY: Cornell University Press, Comstock Publishing Associates, 1997.

Lipinski, M. J., et al. "The Ascent of Cat Breeds: Genetic Evaluations of Breeds and Worldwide Random-bred Populations." *Genomics* 91 (2008): 12–21.

IV. Breed-specific behavioral profiles

The following resources provided much of the methodology for this book.

Hart, B. L. and L. A. Hart. *The Perfect Puppy: How to Choose Your Dog by Its Behavior.* New York: W. H. Freeman and Co., 1988. Reprinted, New York: Barnes & Noble Books, 2001.

Hart, B. L., and M. F. Miller. "Behavioral Profiles of Dog Breeds." *Journal of the American Veterinary Medical Association* 186 (1985): 1175–1180.

V. Why and how cats do that

Why cats purr

Purring is a prominent and mysterious behavior, but little concrete information is available on the whys of purring. The reference below by Peters deals with the mechanism and differences in felid species that do and do not purr. As to the function, an acoustic researcher, Elizabeth von Muggenthaler, first discovered the similarity between the frequency of vibrations in a cat's purring and those used in human physical therapy for promoting wound healing and to reduce swelling and relieve pain.

Peters, G. "Purring and Similar Vocalizations in Mammals." *Mammal Review* 32 (2002): 245–271.

von Muggenthaler, E., and B. Wright. "Solving the Mystery of the Cat's Purr Using the World's Smallest Accelerometer." *Acoustics Australia* 31 (2003): 61.

Why cats yawn

The most prominent theory for yawning, cooling the brain to rev-up the "computer," is profiled by investigators actively working in this field.

Gallup, A. C., and G. G. Gallup. "Yawning and Thermoregulation." *Physiology and Behavior* 95 (2008): 10–16.

Gallup, A. C., and G. G. Gallup. "Yawning as a Brain Cooling Mechanism: Nasal Breathing and Forehead Cooling Diminish the Incidence of Contagious Yawning." *Evolutionary Psychology* 5 (2007): 92–101.

Why cats eat grass and houseplants

The apparent drive that cats and dogs, as carnivores, seem to have to eat plants, especially grass, has been another animal behavior mystery. A strong indication that the behavior could be an instinct of felids and canids living in nature for controlling intestinal parasites comes from observations of chimpanzees. Read more about why cats eat grass and other plants in the following sources.

Hart, B. L. "Why Do Dogs and Cats Eat Grass?" *Veterinary Medicine* 103 (2008): 648–649.

Huffman, M. A., and J. M. Canton. "Self-induced Increase of Gut Motility and the Control of Parasitic Infections in Wild Chimpanzees." *International Journal of Primatology* 22 (2001): 329–346.

Sueda, K. L. C., B. L. Hart, and K. D. Cliff. "Characterisation of Plant Eating in Dogs." *Applied Animal Behaviour Science* 111 (2008): 120–132.

Why cats flip out on catnip

This is a behavior that has no adaptive function; in fact, from the behavioral standpoint, the reaction is downright weird. Nonetheless, many cats seem to enjoy catnip leaves, whether fresh, dry, packaged in a mouse, or loose. The key to understanding the catnip reaction is the geography of the origin of the catnip plant and of the felids that respond to catnip. The following source provides a review of the catnip reaction and the type of plants that evoke it.

Tucker, A. O., and S. S. Tucker. "Catnip and the Catnip Response." *Economic Botany* 42 (1988): 214–231.

Index

141

tive value of, 37; preventing, 19; as territorial marking, 23, 58, 72

veterinarian: as authority, 3–4; questions to ask, 1
vocalization, 3, 40, *41*; gender differences in, 16–18, *17*; predictive value of, 36; quiet breeds, 40, 89; talkative breeds, 40, 93, 107

yawning, 121, 124–26

DISCARD